Hand Reflexology Workbook (Revised)

How to work on someone's hands

Barbara and Kevin Kunz

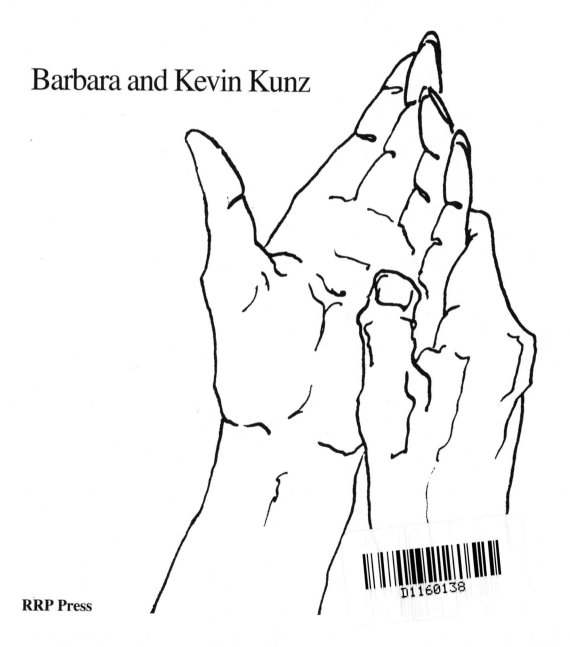

RRP Press

Books by Kevin and Barbara Kunz
• *The Complete Guide To Foot Reflexology* (Revised) (1980/1993)
• *Hand And Foot Reflexology, A Self-help Guide* (Simon & Schuster, 1984)
• *Hand Reflexology Workbook, How to work on someone's hands (Revised)* (1985/ 1999)
• *Medical Applications of Reflexology: Finding in Research About Safety, Efficacy, Mechanism of Action and Cost Effectiveness of Reflexology* (1999)
• *My Reflexologist Says Feet Don't Lie* (2001)
• *Reflexology, Health at your fingertips* (2003 / Dorling Kindersley)

Reflexology Research Project / Kunz Curriculum Systems / RRP Press
P.O. Box 35820, Albuquerque, NM 87176

Find us on the Web:
www.reflexology-research.com
www.foot-reflexologist.com
www.myreflexologist.com

Portions excerpted from:
Hand Reflexology Workbook (Originally published by Prentice Hall, 1985, © 1994 by Kevin and Barbara Kunz)
The Complete Guide to Foot Reflexology (Revised) © 1993 by Kevin and Barbara Kunz
Reflexions, The Journal of Reflexology Research Project © 1980 to1999 by Kevin and Barbara Kunz

10 9 8 7 6 5 4 3 2

Illustrations and book design by Barbara Kunz
Cover art by Camille Young
Cover design by Robert Young

ISBN 0-9606070-4-8

Contents

CHAPTER 1

Consider the Hand

Touch provides a relationship in our lives. It seems to be an element that we seek to add. The stroking of a pet, hug from a loved one, and proverbial pat on the back all speak of the soothing qualities of touch. Touch defines our lives, buffers us from everyday stresses, and soothes the discomforts of illness.

The pursuit of touch as an organized, formalized system is in its infancy. The hands, however, offer an opportunity to exercise activities of our touch sense. The exercise is of pressure and movement with the techniques of reflexology.

The concept of touch as a body activity which can be exercised provides food for thought. Other body activities, such as those of the cardio-vascular system, are the subjects of many exercise programs. While the effect of repetitively practicing the body's activities such as those of the cardio-vascular system are debated, the individuals involved in such programs are a testament to the perception of such exercise as a beneficial pursuit.

The effects of repetitively practicing touch are documented by the individuals who have successfully used reflexology in programs of wellness. Organized touch offers an opportunity to interact with one's quality of life. Results are an individual matter but the pursuit of wellness through touch provides direction and focus for a better life.

Consider the Hand

The hands reach out to touch the world around us, sensing our environment and shaping it to our needs. This ability to manipulate as well as to sense is unique among sensory organs. Hands engage in many activities during the day. Communication is a primary activity. Shaking hands, touching a child, or waving to a friend link us to the world outside. Further communication is possible through the hand's manipulation of writing. Man's written communication has progressed from clay tablet to paper pad to electronic screen. The hand has handled it all.

The hard-working hand has faced its stresses and strains. The repetitive sameness of everyday routines does not often challenge its finely tuned capabilities. In fact, the demand of everyday activities may create a pattern of over-use. To the keyboard operator, the assembly line worker, or anyone whose hands are tools of his or her trade - at work 40 hours a week - the demands of the job create potential for wear and tear.

Indeed, anyone who repetitively practices an activity - even crocheting or tennis - can compensate for potential overuse of the hands by providing variety to fully practice the enormous capabilities of the hands.

Furthermore, the hand, as a part of the survival mechanism communicates with the internal organs. In a fight or flight situation where the body is placed in imminent peril, whole body communication is necessary to ensure survival. The adrenal gland produces needed chemicals, while the hand may reach for a weapon. Instant communication takes place among all body parts.

The roles played by the hand in everyday life are those of manipulator, communicator, and possible defender or befriender. Such activity is possible because of the hand's ability to sense. The sensations are those of pressure, stretch and movement. Consider the handshake, for example. The hand is moved into an appropriate position, stretched out in friendship, and pressure is applied with a firm grip. Pressure, stretch and movement all play a part in this communication.

This manual discusses the application of techniques that replicate the sensation of pressure and movement. The net result of technique application is a soothing addition to the individual's day. The practice of these sensations uses touch as a tool and a respite from stress. Long-term practice becomes a tool of wellness. Those who have used such techniques to work on the hand give us a glimpse of the use of the hands in a program of wellness.

Coping with Life's Stressors

In an attempt to cope with life's stressors, the body adapts. It makes the internal adjustments, creating the physical conditions needed to meet demands. The demands or stressors are those of worry, anxiety, happiness, a snowstorm, a hot day, concrete floors, 90° chairs, and a lifetime of wear and tear. In short, your body itself is a recorded history of what you've done, the environment you've lived in, and how you've felt about the experience.

A stressor is, thus, any demand to which the body must respond. A poke in the eye and a pat on the back both demand attention from the body. Although they are interpreted differently, both are stressors.

Hans Selye, pioneer in stress research, links prolonged stress to stress-related illnesses. He describes stress as a three-stage process. The stress of falling into an icy lake or the stress of a lifetime both follow a pattern of alarm, adaptation/resistance, and exhaustion. The phases are alarm (an immediate response), adaptation (a more or less balanced state of resistance), and exhaustion (a breakdown of resistance).

Stress is the process of meeting the world around us. Adapting to the demands made upon us is an on-going process. Like any other process, it is an improvable skill. **The ability to best adapt to stress is a matter of knowing what to request from your body.** It is possible to make a request for the best possible adaptation under the circumstances. A request to interrupt the pattern of stress provides a break in the routine, resolving the wear-and-tear aspect of continuous stress.

Speaking the Body's Language to Counter Stress

The best possible adaptation to stress is the interruption of it, the practice of something different. Sensory signals such as sight, taste, touch, smell, pressure, stretch, and movement are the sensory components necessary for the organized activity of movement. These key sensory signals offer an opportunity to communicate with the body in its own language.

An infant struggling to stand demonstrates the learning and practice of an activity that we as adults take for granted. The ability to move through the world and handle it is an ability that is practiced and occurs unconsciously on a continuous basis throughout the day. Lifting oneself from the chair and walking across the room is an example of a physical event that requires little or no thought of the muscular interaction required. The routine involved in such an activity is below the awareness level, because each detail would occupy every waking moment if each step had to be throughout.

Automatically, however, as we move specifics are measured, indicating pressure, stretch and movement such as resistance. Imagine the activities of the hand in moving a couch down a flight of stairs: pushing, pulling, lifting, gripping, or perhaps, praying may be involved. All require measured response, translating intention into action.

To be able to move, the body must "see" itself. Such perception requires information about muscles, tendons and joints. From such information, the body creates a picture of itself. The messengers of self-perception are those that apprise the body of pressure, stretch and movement - the proprioceptors. Proprioception means literally, "to perceive oneself." The exercise of such perception is the subject of this manual.

Proprioceptors are sophisticated gauges in the muscles, tendons and joints. Just as the thermostat measures heat, proprioceptors measure the hand's activities. They report on whether the hand is open, closed, carrying weight, writing a letter, or shooting baskets. Everyday activities seldom call for the full practice of proprioceptive potential. The techniques of reflexology offer the possibility of exercise for fine-tuning capabilities of the hands.

The reflexologist thus provides to the client an exercise of proprioception. This exercise provides interruption of stress as well as conditioning and education for the body as a whole. Clients goals are achieved as the body makes a better adaptation to stress.

The Body's Relationships Applied

The basic principle of working with the body in its own language is that work on one part of the body influences another part. One part of the body relates to another and establishes a body relationship. The relationships have a basis to the body's response to demand or stress. For example, in response to standing up, the body aligns itself to gravity. To meet the demand a longitudinal relationship, that of zones, is established among body parts.

Organization by Stride

Stride, or the ability to walk, is a coordinated activity of all body parts, including the hands. Balancing on a log to cross a stream, for example, calls for the participation of the hands. A similar participation is involved in every footstep. Thus, the hands are linked in the body's communication system.

The communication necessary to walk and perform the hands' tasks of handling, manipulating and carrying involves stretch. Stretch apprises the body of which muscles are working and which are relaxing. When one muscle contracts, another muscle relaxes. An extremely stretched muscle is opposed by a corresponding relaxed muscle.

Organization by Movement

The demands of movement create a relationship between body parts. Coordination is necessary to achieve purposeful movement. Body parts must work together. For example, although a tennis racket is held in the hand, the entire body coordinates its activities to achieve the goal of hitting the ball with the racket. The hand participates in many coordinated activities during the day. Whether swinging a hammer, writing a letter, or playing the piano, the hands work with the body to move through the day.

The Learning Process

Pressure, stretch, and movement are requests in the body's own language. These signals essentially ask the body to interrupt its present programming and pay attention to their request. The request is one for change, an interruption in stress. To make body language and body relationships work for you, apply the same elements as you would in any learning situation. The elements are a focused learning effort, practice, comparing and contrasting. In this manner, one builds a body of experience and a body of knowledge. Reflexology techniques are a learning experience. The skill developed is the ability to interrupt stress to form a program of wellness.

In learning, practice, consistency and frequency play a role. Consider learning how to type. One practices every few days for a certain period of time to become a proficient typist. Investing more time and effort in practicing improves one' skills. The techniques of reflexology are applied on a similar basis. Pressure, stretch and/or movement is practiced on a consistent and frequent basis. The amount of time spent practicing influences the results.

Just as a basketball team focuses its learning efforts with a series of drills, body language focuses its learning around a pattern of technique application and the body relationships. A purposeful pattern of pressure, for example, establishes a method for exercising the pressure sensors of the whole hand.

The body actually learns by comparing and contrasting. The practitioner compares the current hand to other hands on which he or she has worked. The hand being worked contrasts the before and after of technique application.

In summary, to make body language and body relationships work for you, apply the same elements as you would in any other learning situation. One's influence on the body is a result of careful consideration of how the body works.

In Summary

• What is hand reflexology? Hand reflexology is the physical act of applying specific pressure techniques to the hands with an assessment based on reflexology areas and zones.

• How does hand reflexology work? In hand reflexology, pressure techniques are applied to the hand to interrupt stress.

• Why does hand reflexology work? Hand reflexology works by communication with the body in its own language and providing a break in the pattern of stress.

Why work on the hands? The hands provide access to the body and its internal organs, because of the need for the whole body to respond in times of danger. In the fight or flight response to danger, the internal organs prepare for either eventuality; the feet ready themselves to take a stand or flee and the hands reach for a weapon or participate in flight. Reflexology takes advantage of this mechanism. The hands and feet, like a computer keyboard, are a way to feed information in.

How does an individual benefit from hand reflexology? Hand reflexology provides an opportunity to exercise the body by interrupting patterns of stress. There always exists a possibility for change though the application of positive actions.

Reflexology techniques are tools used in programs of wellness.

We've seen people use these tools in a myriad of ways as a means of taking action in response to their own needs. The painter whose aging hands were failing, the computer operator whose hands were exhausted, a senior citizen who used his hands to speed recovery from an operation - all became involved and gained control.

A variety of benefits has been derived from the use of these tools. The greatest benefit, however, may be the opportunity for positive action - active involvement in addressing the situation.

What is the benefit to me of working on other peoples' hands? Working on other people's hands is a mechanism to interact with other people. From the concerned family member to the professional reflexologist, we've seen the creative use of pressure, stretch and movement in work with others. The benefit is in providing others with these sensory experiences: break in the routine to cope with stress, an approach to a health problem, a nonthreatening touch tool. Hand reflexology techniques provide a means to work with each situation.

CHAPTER 2

Reflexology: Charts

Organization in Reflexology by Chart and Function

Organization by Zone

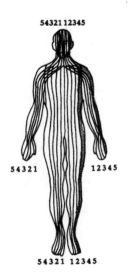

Zones recognize the relationship between gravity and the upright body. Zones are a system for organizing the various parts of the body. They can be thought of as guidelines, or markers, that link one part to another.

There are ten equal longitudinal zones running the length of the body from the top of the head to the tips of the toes. The number ten corresponds to the number of fingers and toes and therefore provides a convenient numbering system. Each finger and each toe falls into one zone, with the left thumb, for example, occurring in the same zone as the left big toe and so on.

Using the zonal chart, trace the ten zones on your own body.

Begin with your feet and trace imaginary lines from each toe up the leg, through the trunk of the body to the top of the head. Each toe represents a zone. Do the same exercise with the hands. Begin tracing from each finger. Note on the chart how the numbered zones intersect with each other in the neck and head area.

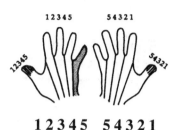

A portion of the hand relates to a longitudinal section of the body. For example, the portion of the hand indicated relates to the section of the body indicated. Note that one half of the head is represented by the thumb of each hand. Each thumb represents five zones.

Organization by Reiteration

Reiteration is a relationship in which the body whole is reflected on a body par. In reflexology, the body whole is reiterated on the hands and feet. As applied to the hands, reiteration recognizes the relationship between the whole body, hands, and the need for survival.

To visualize the body on the hands, note the illustrations. Each hand represents half of the body (right hand = right side; left hand = left side). The spine itself is divided in half, with each hand having a spinal area along the inside edge. To represent a whole body on the hands, the hands are placed side by side with the palms down.

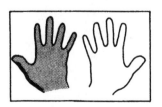

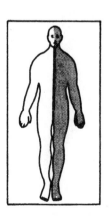

15

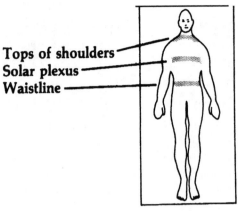

Tops of shoulders
Solar plexus
Waistline

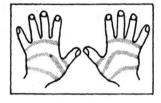

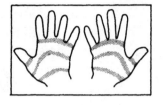

Lateral zones establish guidelines to aid in comparison between the body and hands.

The representation on the hands of a part of the body may be located using these guides. For example, the left shoulder is represented on the hands in an area between the lateral zones, tops of shoulders, and solar plexus. This portion of the hand includes representations of the front, back, and internal sections of the body. The top side of the hand is a further representation of these same sections.

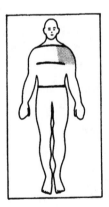

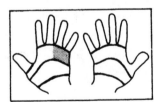

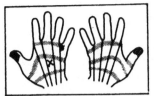 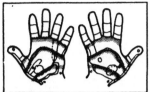 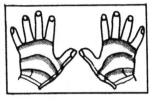 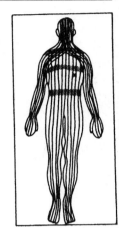

The lateral and longitudinal zones form a grid system, which establishes a more detailed locating system. For example, to locate on the hands the portion of the body indicated, the zone is traced to the hand. The lateral markers indicate boundary lines within which the final location is determined.

With the grid system as a basis, a reiteration of the body's internal organs is reflected on the hands. A comparison of the foot and hand reflexology charts shows the same reflex area pattern with differences due to the anatomical structures of the foot and hand.

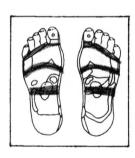 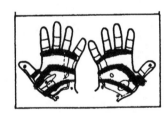

The length of the fingers and thumb as compared to the toes creates one difference. The smaller carpal bones and heel of the hand as contrasted to the foot's tarsal bones and heel creates another. The webbings of the hand creates distinctive areas on the hands as contrasted to the foot. The results of these anatomical differences include an expanded neck reiterative pattern, a smaller pattern of reflex areas below the waistline, and the unique webbings.

There is an exception to the rule that the right hand equals the right side of the body and the left hand equals the left side of the body and vice versa. Any problem involving the head area crosses over to the opposite thumb for emphasis.

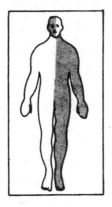

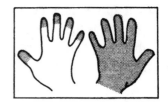

Organization by Referral

Referral relationships offer an additional means to relate body parts, specifically the limbs. The relationship is based on zones. Following the basic premise, one segment of a zone affects and is affected by any other segment of the zone. Thus, a segment of zone one in the arm relates to a segment of zone one in the leg. The shoulder relates to the hip, the upper arm to the thigh, the elbow to the knee, the forearm to the calf, the wrist to the ankle, the hand to the foot.

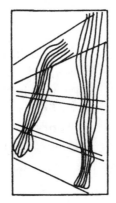

shoulder	**hip**
upper arm	**thigh**
elbow	**knee**
forearm	**calf**
wrist	**ankle**
hand	**foot**

The foot relates to the hand zone by zone and (almost) bone by bone. The first zone of the hand corresponds to the first zone of the foot and so forth. The first phalanx of the hand relates to the first phalanx of the foot. The distal phalanx of the first metacarpal relates to the distal phalanx of the first metatarsal. The first metatarsal of the foot relates to the first metacarpal of the hand and so forth. The carpal bones correspond to the tarsal bones.

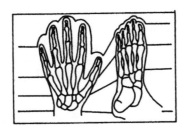

CHAPTER 3

Professional Issues

As a reflexologist, you signal your professionalism through what you say, do, and display in the workplace. What you say and do demonstrates you mastery of professional skills. You want the individual to feel safe in your hands, that you are well qualified, and that this is a service he or she values. Preparation is required to reflect a credible professional image. In reflexology this includes the consideration of basic professional issues.

Laws, Rules and Regulations

Two types of laws apply to hand reflexology practice: (1) business licensing and (2) licensing of other professionals. Business licensing is required by a business of cities. The general issue is one of taxation and zoning. Not all business are allowed to operate in any zoned area. To ascertain business licensing and zoning requirements, contact the appropriate department of the city government, usually the taxation and revenue department.

In some cities and states of the United States, the provider of reflexology services is required to obtain licensing for the profession of massage therapy. To ascertain massage therapy licensing requirements, contact the appropriate department of the city government, usually the taxation and revenue department and of the state government. The state may regulate through a regulation and licensing department or an education department.

Do not diagnose, prescribe, or treat for specific illness

The reflexologist is also subject to the medical practices acts that define the role of the medical professional. In general, it is noted that the reflexologist does not infringe on the medical profession by diagnosing, prescribing, and treating for specific illnesses.

The role of the reflexologist is to apply techniques based on certain ideas. The presentation of these ideas by the professional practitioner — one who accepts money for his or her services — should be handled with care. The basic rule is always talk in general terms; never specifically address a problem. Assessment and evaluation in reflexology are a reflection of the body whole. While the vocabulary of assessment in reflexology is based on body parts, such as kidney or liver, such assessment has the potential for being misconstrued as the making of a diagnosis or the practice of medicine without a license. Do not diagnose, prescribe, or treat for a specific illness.

What Reflexology Does

In reflexology, assessment is made by observation (primarily, of what the thumb feels). Observation is categorized as, for example, a kidney reiterative area. By using terms such as "kidney reflex area, the practitioner further emphasizes his or her awareness of the service offered by reflexology.

Reflexology is the practice of sensory signals, the exercise of the hand's potential. Such practice is based on certain causal relationships. These causal relationships are not the same as those used by the traditional medical community in the diagnosis of a medical problem.

The sensory assessment garnered by the reflexologist is a reflection of the body whole and the demands made upon it. The demands are those of walking upright and acting in relationship to gravity. The goal in the application of technique is the exercise of the sensors that make weight-carrying and manipulation possible. The important assessment is the one made by the body as a sensory technique is applied. A picture is provided to the body from which judgments are made. Judgments are in the body's language of muscle tension, among others.

Do Not Work on an Undiagnosed Problem

An undiagnosed problem is a problem that is acute enough to cause the client concern but which has not yet been examined by a physician. For example, a painful finger may be an injured finger that needs medical care. When in doubt, refer the client to medical personnel. Failure to refer to appropriate medical care is the chief concern of legal authorities about alternative health in general.

The Working Reflexologist

Working Position

The optimal working situation for a hand reflexology session should include accommodation for the client's comfort, such as a soft working surface for the client's hand, and the reflexologist's comfort. A pillow or a folded towel serves as both a padded surface on which to work and an area of activity.

In the ideal situation, the client sits stretched back and relaxed in a recliner with hand resting on a pillow or towel placed on the arm rest. The reflexologist sits alongside in a stenographer or other chair with wheels. It is easiest if the reflexologist sits to the right hand side of the client when applying work to the right hand and to the left hand side of the client when applying work to the left hand. Reaching across the client to work the opposite hand can be awkward and uncomfortable. Client and reflexologist may also sit face to face over a narrow table with the client's hand resting on a towel or pillow, or, client and reflexologist may sit side by side.

Hand Etiquette

When working with hands, consider yourself to be politely yet firmly in control of the hand being worked on. There is some difficulty in picking up another person's hand to work on because of the cultural uneasiness of "hand-holding." To counter this demands the thoughtful development of hand courtesy so that the practitioner may work in a professional manner. To give further indication of control, keep at least one of your hands on the hand of the person on whom you are working. Continuity is thus established.

For example, signify the beginning and end of a session with phrases that indicate you are starting and finishing. The phrase "May I have your hand?" can serve as notification that the session is beginning. The phrase "I am finished — you may have your hand back" signals the end of a session. A further indication of the conclusion of the session is to return the hand to a resting position in closer proximity to the client. Should any interruption arise during the session, the same beginning and ending phrases may be used.

At the start of the session, ask the client to remove any rings, bracelets or a watch that may interfere with your work. Have a bowl or basket available in which to place jewelry during the session.

Safety Issues

Communicable diseases are spread through the ingestion (eating or drinking) or inhalation (breathing) of bacteria or virus organisms or their toxins. This may occur either directly or indirectly. Many disease-causing organisms are commonly found in the intestinal tract, oral cavity, and nose of both ill and healthy persons. Illness occurs when these organisms are transferred to other persons or when they are transferred to another site in the body. Examples of direct transmission include instances in which an infected person (carrier) coughs or spits and airborne organisms are the inhaled by nearby persons, or when an infected person fails to wash the hands following urination or defecation and organisms are transmitted by touching another individual and that person ingests the organisms. Direct transmissions may also occur when organisms are transferred from an infected skin lesion or dirty hands to an open cut in the skin.

An example of indirect transmission is that which occurs when an infected person fails to wash their hands following urination or defecation and then prepares food. The organisms are transferred to the food, where they may multiply and produce toxins. When the food is ingested by others, the disease is transmitted. Indirect transmission also occurs when sewage-contaminated shellfish are eaten, or when waste-contaminated water is ingested.

Washing Your Hands

Washing your hands before and between sessions is a necessity. It assures the client of cleanliness and a professional approach in the prevention of communicable disease.

According to public health professionals, hand washing, when done correctly, is one of the most effective ways of preventing the spread of communicable diseases. Good hand washing technique is easy to learn and can significantly reduce the spread of infectious diseases in both children and adults.

Hands should be thoroughly washed following coughing, sneezing, rubbing the nose or defecation. Proper hand washing can effectively reduce the incidence of illnesses such as staphylococcus infections, salmonelosis, typhoid fever, influenza, and the common cold. It should be noted that this is effective in reducing illness for both the reflexologists and client.

What is an effective hand washing technique?
There is more to hand washing than you think! By rubbing your hands vigorously with soapy water, you pull the dirt plus the oily soils free from your skin. The soap lather suspends both the dirt and germs trapped inside and are then quickly washed away.

Follow these four simple steps to keeping hands clean:
1. Wet your hands with warm running water.

2. Add soap, then rub your hands together, making a soapy lather. Do this away from the running water for at least 10 seconds, being careful not to wash the lather away. Wash the front and back of your hands, as well as between your fingers and under your nails.

(According to the CDC, the specific hand washing procedure consists of 6 steps of ten seconds duration and five strokes per step: (1) palm to palm, (2) palm over dorsum, (3) palm to palm, fingers interlaced, (4) back of fingers to opposing palms, (5) rotate thumb in palm and (6) rotate fingers in palm. Repeat steps 2, 4, 5, and 6 with the other hand.)

3. Rinse your hands well under warm running water. Let the

water run back into the sink, not down to your elbows. Turn off the sink with a paper towel and dispose in a proper receptacle.

4. Dry hands thoroughly with a clean towel.

What type of soap should be used?

Any type of soap may be used. However, bar soap should be kept in a self draining holder that is cleaned thoroughly before new bars are put out and liquid soap containers (which must be used in day care centers) should be used until empty and cleaned before refilling. To prevent chapping use a mild soap with warm water, pat rather than rub hands dry, and apply lotion liberally and frequently.

What are some things I should avoid regarding hand washing?

DON'T use a standing basin of water to rinse hands.

DON'T use a common hand towel. Always use disposable towels.

DON'T use sponges or non-disposable cleaning cloths unless you launder them on a regular basis, adding chlorine bleach to the wash water. Remember that germs thrive on moist surfaces!

The Visual Inspection

Before working, briefly inspect the client's hands for cuts, rashes or injuries. Avoid cuts or injuries by placing a bandage over the area to make the session as safe as possible.

Ask the client if any part of the hand should be avoided. With older clients be aware of the potential for painful enlarged, red or arthritic finger joints.

The AIDS Question

Research has shown that there is no potential for the spread of AIDS through skin contact. There is a problem, however, with blood to blood contact, exposure of an open wound to an open wound on another individual. There is a general rule of thumb for reflexologists that any breach in the skin is covered with a bandage and is to be avoided. The reflexologist should be aware of any breaches in his or her skin that could become exposed.

Use a common sense approach to such concerns. Keep bandages in your workplace so that you can provide one to any client to cover any open wound on his or her hand. Carefully consider your own work if you have an open cut or rash on your own hands.

Amount of Pressure

The client's comfort level is the primary determinant of the amount of pressure to be exerted. Tastes in applied pressure vary from client to client. To establish an individual client's preference, ask the client to indicate discomfort due to the pressure exerted. Some clients may even request additional pressure. The goal of the practitioner is to stay within the client's comfort zone.

Respect an Individual's Response to Pain

Pain is not an activity that needs to be practiced. There is a difference between a client's comment of, "It hurts good" and one of "It hurts." One method of eliciting comments on the amount of pressure preferred by the client is to ask, "Will you tell me if the pressure is too much?" This is an especially appropriate question when applying techniques to areas you think might be sensitive; for example, working with the pancreas reiterative area of a diabetic.

Fingernail Length

The nails of the reflexologist's walking finger and thumb should not make contact with the skin of the hand at any time.

Duration of a Hand Reflexology Workout

A thorough workout may last 30 to 45 minutes.

Instruments

In reflexology, instruments are utilized as self-help tools. Control and leverage in the application of techniques are the tools of the practitioner. Instruments that have no feeling have no place as practitioner's tools. The easiest way to pursue safe, effective techniques is with your own hand.

Creams, Lotions and Goo

Creams, lotions, and oils are tools of hand massage. While hand massage is a valid practice in itself, it is not the same as hand reflexology. The techniques of reflexology require friction between the walking thumb and the skin of the hand. Use of creams, lotions, and oils at the end of a session is an individual practitioner decision. Note, however, that the practitioner's hands become covered with the cream, lotion or oil and their presence will be a factor in the session with the following client.

The Role of the Reflexologist as an Advocate of Self-Help

Self-help is the involvement of the client in his or her own program of wellness. Reflexology provides technique application that is an opportunity to practice and exercise the hand's capabilities. As in any exercise program, time spent exercising the hand is a factor in the program. The addition of the client's self-help program is an opportunity to spend more time exercising. (See *Hand and Foot Reflexology, A Self-Help Guide,* Kevin and Barbara Kunz, Prentice-Hall, Inc., 1984.)

CHAPTER 4

Anatomy/Physiology

Anatomy is the structure of an organism or body. Physiology is the branch of biology dealing with the functions and vital processes of living organisms. Disease is the dysfunction of a portion of the structure or function of the body. To understand the basis of hand function and dysfunction, an understanding of names of hand parts and intended functions of those parts is helpful. For these reasons a study of anatomy and physiology is useful for the hand reflexology student.

For example, the common hand malady of carpal tunnel syndrome is known to many of us by name. Carpal tunnel syndrome illustrates what happens when several anatomical parts and physiological functions become disrupted. Repeated demands on specific parts of the body lead to physical damage. In the case of carpal tunnel syndrome, the physical act of typing, for example, combines with body positioning and job stress to result in inability to function. Specifically, a major nerve of the hand is compressed as it passes through a narrow "tunnel" of bone and ligament at the wrist.

In the language of anatomy and physiology, what has happened is that "repetitive stress injury" has taken place as the "median nerve" becomes compressed due to swelling of the "flexor tendons" and the "transverse carpal ligament" as the nerve passes through the "carpal tunnel." A basic knowledge of anatomy enables one to translate this explanation into a cause and effect rationale that can lead to helping the individual impacted by, for example, carpal tunnel syndrome. In addition, the medical community exchanges information in such precise terms to communicate concisely and accurately with other professionals.

As we work through anatomical terms and physiological processes, keep in mind that the functioning and dysfunctioning of the structures and processes described in anatomy and physiology speak to impact on real humans.

By the way, the translation of carpal tunnel syndrome is that the median nerve conveys sensation to the hand from the rest of the body. It passes through a narrow opening at the wrist, so called the carpal tunnel in recognition of the eight small carpal bones in the heel of the hand. The flexor tendons which also pass through the narrow opening attach the muscles that enable the hand to flex or move toward the forearm. The transverse carpal ligament joins bone to bone, connecting the bone at the base of the thumb to bone at the base of the little finger. It thus transverses the carpal bones and forms a tunnel for nerves and tendons.

The Hand

The hand is the most versatile part of the skeleton. It enables people to grasp and manipulate objects. It is capable of weight carrying functions and has extensive sensory capabilities. Take a moment to consider what makes this possible. To lift one's little finger, for example, the desire to do so must first (unconsciously) be originate a nd be generated by the brain. The message is then conveyed through a complex of nerves to the little finger. It is a message conveyed to tendons and muscles which will make the movement possible. The message specifically recognizes in what position the little finger rests before it is instructed to move. After all, if the fingers of the hand are formed into a tight fist, the instructions will be different from those directed to a hand positioned with outstretched fingers.

Consider now the act of holding this book or typing or writing or any one of the many complicated activities our hands perform. The how and why these actions take place is the subject of this chapter.

Complex and intricate hand movements are achieved by using the small muscles that are contained entirely within the hand and the much larger forearm muscles. A common perception is that the arm below the elbow has no reason for its existence other than to move the hand. While the intrinsic muscles of the hand perform many functions, many activities of the hand take place thanks to the muscles and tendons of the forearm. Consider for a moment the action of the thumb during the application of thumb walking technique. Observe the forearm of your working arm as you apply thumb walking technique to your other forearm. Note the activity of muscles in the forearm in moving the thumb. Because of this relationship, this chapter will include information about both the hand and forearm.

Terms of Position, Direction and Action

In studying anatomical terminology, it is helpful to understand that the same words are used again and again in a variety of anatomical terms and that it is the combinations of these words that create specific anatomical terms. For example, the word **dorsal** refers to toward the back of the body in general. The word is used specifically in the phrase "dorsal surface of the hand" to refer to the top, finger side of the hand.

Common terms of anatomical position and direction

Certain terms are used in anatomy to aid in the visualization of body parts, describing the relationship of one part to another:

• **Anterior** or **ventral** refers a structure toward the front or in front of the body. The anterior surface or ventral surface of the body is the front of the body or towards the front.

• **Posterior** or **dorsal** refers to a structure more toward the back of the body or in the back of the body. The posterior surface or dorsal surface is the back of the body or towards the back.

• **Medial** refers to a structure more towards the middle or median plane of the body. The belly button is medial to the hip bone.

• **Lateral** refers to a structure away from the median plane. The hip bone is lateral to the belly button.

• **Proximal** refers to the limbs, closer to the median plane. The first segment of the thumb closest to the body of the hand is called proximal.

• **Distal** refers to the limbs, away from the median plane. The second segment of the thumb further away from the body of the hand is called distal.

• **Superficial** refers to on the surface. In the following discussion, some muscles are referred to as superficial, noting their position toward the surface.

• **Deep** refers to below the surface. Some muscles are deep muscles, below the surface.

Terms of position and direction of the hands:

Specifically in reference to the hand:

• The palm or **palmar surface** is the anterior (ventral) or flexor surface of the hand from wrist to fingers.

• The **dorsal surface** is the topside of the hand from wrist to fingers.

• The **medial surface** is toward the little finger side of the body. Think of the standing human figure with the palmar surface of the hand turned toward you, the little finger resting against the body.

• The **lateral surface** is toward the thumb side of the hand. Again, think of the standing figure with the palmar surface turned, the thumb resting away further from the median of the body than the little finger side.

Bones of the Hand

Of the 200 to 210 bones in the human body, 54 are in the hands, 27 in each one. Bone is living tissue, growing and changing throughout life. Throughout childhood, cartilage turns into bone in a regular sequence. Bones are given rigidity and hardness by minerals such as calcium. Bone will give up its minerals in times of shortage when other parts of the body need them more. All through life, bone is continually being reconstructed and reshaped as a result of the stresses, bends, and breaks it endures. A bone is one-third water with blood vessels supplying oxygen and nutrients and carrying away waste. Bones have nerves that feel pain and pressure.

The bones of the hands are referred to in general terms as: the bones of the wrist, the carpals; the long straight bones of the palm, the metacarpals, and fingers, the phalanges. The twenty-seven bones of the hand are ingeniously arranged for function. The fourteen **phalanges** are arranged in jointed continuous segments that enable independent or united action. Bony support is provided to the palm of the hand by five **metacarpal** bones (one for each digit). The eight **carpal** bones form the heel of the hand and interface with the bones of the forearm to create the wrist.

The general terms of position and direction for the body carry over to the naming of the bones of the fingers. The fingers consist of three bones each, individually called a **phalanx**. Each of the three is named for its proximity to the body of the hand. The bone most distant from the body is the **distal phalanx**. That in the center is the **middle phalanx**. The bone of the finger closest to the hand is the **proximal phalanx**. The thumb consists of two bones, a distal phalanx and a proximal phalanx.

Phalanges

Metacarpals

Carpals

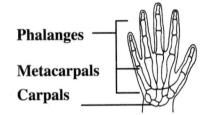

The phalanges are referred to by number beginning with the thumb as the first phalange and the little finger as the fifth. Thus the **first proximal phalanx** is the bone of the thumb closest to the body of the hand. The **right first proximal phalanx** is on the right hand.

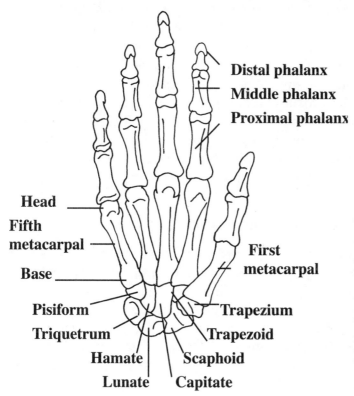

Distal phalanx
Middle phalanx
Proximal phalanx

Head
Fifth metacarpal
Base
Pisiform
Triquetrum
Hamate
Lunate
First metacarpal
Trapezium
Trapezoid
Scaphoid
Capitate

Palmar Surface

The five metacarpal bones are referred to by number. The **first metacarpal** refers to the palmar bone below the thumb, the second metacarpal refers to the palmar bone below the index finger and so forth with the fifth metacarpal in the palm below the little finger. The **metacarpal head** refers to the part of the metacarpal bone proximal to the phalanges. The **base of the metacarpal** refers to the part of the bone closest to the carpal bones. The **right first metacarpal** refers to the right hand.

The eight carpal bones are roughly arranged in two rows of four each. The **scaphoid, lunate, triquetrum,** and **pisiform** fan across the heel of the hand from below the thumb to the little finger respectively. These four bones interface with the bones of the forearm and form the wrist. The **trapezuim, trapezoid, capitate,** and **hamate** form a second tier of carpal bones ranging across the heel of the hand from thumb to little finger respectively.

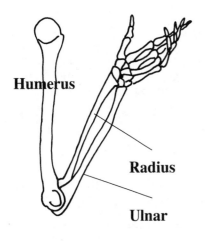

Humerus

Radius

Ulnar

The Bones of the Forearm

The forearm consists of two bones, the **radius** and the **ulna**. The radius spans the forearm from the elbow to the wrist below the thumb. It is wider at the wrist and, with the carpal bones, forms the wrist. The ulna bone stabilizes the forearm. It is wider at the elbow, where it forms a hinge-type joint. Rotation of the radius at the elbow rotates the forearm, wrist and hand without moving the ulna. To observe this action, hold your hand out. Now, move your hand into position as if to type with palmar surface down. This was accomplished by rotation of the radius bones

The joints of the forearm and hands

A **joint** is a point of juncture between two bones. "Joints because of their location and constant use, are prone to stress, injuries, and inflammation. The main diseases affecting the joints are rheumatic fever, rheumatoid arthritis, osteoarthritis, and gout. Injuries are contusions, sprains, dislocations and penetrating wounds." *Taber's Cyclopedic Medical Dictionary*, F. A. Davis Co., New York, 1981

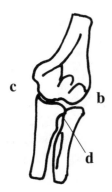

c

b

d

The anatomical names of joints reflect the names of the bones that intersect. The wrist is formed at the point where the radius bone meets the carpal bones. The wrist is thus called the **radiocarpal joint (a)**. See below. The elbow is comprised of three joints: the **humero-ulnar (b)**, where the humerus (large bone of the upper arm) meets the ulna of the forearm; the **radio-humeral (c)**, where the radius meets the humerus, and the **radio-ulnar (d)**, where the radius and the ulnar meet.

The joints of the hand are similarly named. Joints between the segments of the fingers, the phalanges, are named **interphalangeal joints**. **(e)** The joints where the long metacarpal bones meet the phalanges are named **metacarpophalangeal joints (f)**. The joints between the metacarpals are **intermetacarpal joints (g)**. The joints between the metacarpal bones and the carpal bones are the **carpometacarpal joints (h)**. The joints between carpal bones are the **intercarpal joints (i)**.

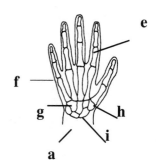

Terms describing action of the fingers and wrist

Four basic anatomical terms describe the actions of the body. **Adduction** is the movement of a limb toward the midline of the body. Think in terms of moving your fingers together. Try it. **Abduction** is the movement of a limb away from the midline. Think in terms of spreading your fingers. Try it. **Flexing** is a body part that bends upon itself. Think of bending the finger to curl it. Try it. **Extension** is the opposite of flexion, bringing members of a limb into or toward a straight condition. Think of uncurling your fingers and stretching them back. Try it.

These words are also used in phrase to describe actions of the fingers. As you have practiced the above you have participated in **finger adduction**, **finger abduction**, **finger flexion**, and **finger extension**.

Major muscles of the hand

"Intricate hand movements are achieved by using the small muscles that are contained entirely within the hand (the **intrinsic muscles**), and the much larger forearm muscles. The forearm muscles are connected to the bones of the hand by long tendons. Tendons and ligaments are often confused with one another. A **tendon** is the fibrous attachment of a muscle to a bone. A **ligament** is a fibrous attachment between bones." (http://www.letsfindout.com/subjects/body/handmmov.html) An example of a ligament is the transverse carpal ligament that connects two of the carpal bones to form the carpal tunnel.

Hand muscles are referred to as **'intrinsic'** if they are entirely inside the parameters of the hand. Of particular importance in movement of the hand is a group of muscles responsible for the movements of the thumb. The movements of the thumb comprise 50% of the hand's activities. Of note is the thumb's ability to work in opposition to the fingers. This anatomical feature in itself creates humankind's ability to use tools.

The actions of the thumb take place with the activity of three muscles referred to as the thenar eminence. The **thenar eminence (a, b, c)** is the bulge in the palm of the hand below the thumb, the **pollex**.

Wrist actions are described in a similar manner. In **wrist adduction**, the hand is moved outward at the little finger side. (It is envisioned that the body is standing with the hands by the sides, palm side up. In wrist adduction, the hand is moved toward the midline of the body which is thus the little finger side.) **Wrist abduction** moves the hand outward at the thumb side. **Wrist flexion** causes the palm of the hand to move toward the forearm. A **wrist extension** causes the dorsal surface of the hand to move toward the forearm.

The names of the three muscles reflect the action of the thumb made possible and location (**pollicis**). The **opponens pollicus (a)** muscle makes possible the movement of the thumb in opposition to the fingers. This ability makes possible grasping, manipulation, and tool use. Holding a piece of paper, gripping a pen or working with a screw drive are all made possible by the opposition of thumb and fingers. Bring your thumb and index finger together. Your opponens pollicis made this happen.

Move your thumb away from the body of your hand. Your **abductor pollicis brevis** (b) was at work. Bring your thumb toward the center of your hand (in air, not touching). The **flexor pollicis brevis** (c) was at work. Now circle your thumb in the air. The three muscles of the thenar eminence work together to create the thumb's unique movement of circumduction (turnings a circle). Adduction, bringing the thumb up against the hand, is made possible by a deep muscle, the **adductor pollicis** (d).

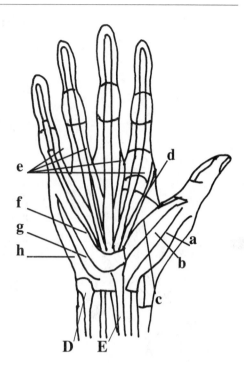

The muscles of the fingers themselves make possible the flexing or extension of the fingers. Other deep muscles make possible certain movements of the fingers. Deep in the body of the hand, the **palmar interosseus** muscles make possible the adduction of the fingers. The **palmar and dorsal interosseus** muscles make it possible to abduct and adduct certain digits (buried deep in the palm of the hand, lengthwise between metacarpal bones). The **lumbricals (e)** works with the interosseus to flex and extend certain joints.

The muscles of the **hypothenar eminence (f, g, h)** move the fifth digit, the little finger. This is important to oppositional grasping. The muscles of the hypothenar eminence work with those of the thenar eminence in a complementary fashion. These muscles are the **opponens digiti minimi (f), the flexor digiti minimi (g), and the abductor digiti minimi (h)**.

Major Muscles of the Forearm

Major muscles of the forearm are extrinsic muscles that create flexing and extending movements of the wrist and hand

The **flexors** of the wrist (carpus) and the fingers (digits) lie as muscles in deep layer, intermediate layer and superficial layer. They are:

flexor digitorum profundus (H)
flexor digitorum superficialis (G)
flexor carpi ulnaris (D)
palmaris longus (E)
flexor carpi radialis (F)

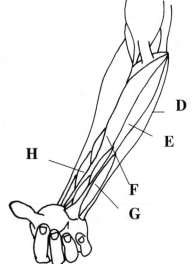

The **extensors** of the wrist, hand and fingers are:

extensor carpi ulnaris (J)
extensor digit minimi (K)
extensor digitorum (L)
extensor indicis (M)
extensor carpi radialis longus (N)
extensor carpi radialis brevis (O)

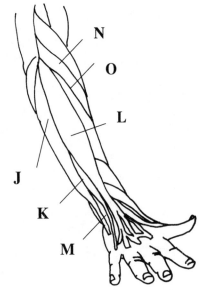

Forearm muscles acting on the thumb include:

abductor pollicis longus (P)
extensor pollicis brevis (Q)
adductor pollicis longus (R)

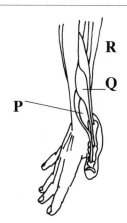

Nerves and Dermatomes of the Hands

Major nerves

Nerves connect with various parts of the hand and forearm to make movement and sensation possible. Three main nerves travel to the hand. The **median nerve (X)** supplies sensation to part of the forearm, the thenar muscles, the thumb and two and a half fingers. The **ulnar nerve** (Y) supplies areas of the forearm and most intrinsic muscles of the hand. The **radial nerve** (Z) supplies muscles of the upper arm and muscles of the forearm that create extension of the wrist and hand.

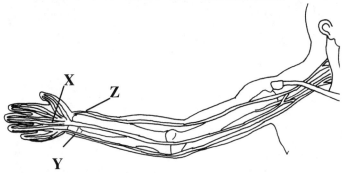

These three nerves actually project (originate) from the spinal cord. Injury or stress on these nerves can be caused by impingement at the projection from the point of origin by the vertebrae of the spine. These nerves originate at the spinal cord and pass through the vertebrae of the spine at the fifth, sixth, seventh, and eighth cervical vertebrae as well as the first thoracic vertebrae. Stress on the neck is thus of importance in influence of sensation into the forearm, hands and fingers.

Dermatome

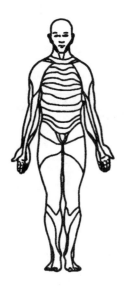

The term dermatome refers to an area of skin innervated by a single spinal nerve (sensory nerve). Each is termed a dermatome. Dermatomes of the fifth, sixth, seventh, eighth cervical, and first thoracic vertebrae innervate the arms and hands.

Nerve receptors

The hands receive sensory information through two types of nerve receptors. The **exteroceptors** transmit information from the body's surface about touch, tactile sensation, temperature, pressure and pain to the spinal cord and brain for interpretation and response. The **proprioceptors** respond to information received from within the body, responding to pressure, position or stretch.

Circulatory System of the Hands

The major arteries of the forearm and hand, carrying blood from the heart, are the radial and the ulnar, named for the bones they parallel. The superficial palmer arch, palmer digital and deep palmer arch feed the hand itself. The major veins, carrying blood away from the hand and forearm are the dorsal digital and network, basilic, median vein of the forearm, cephalic and the median cubital.

Disorders of the Hands

Carpal Tunnel Syndrome

Carpal tunnel syndrome is a condition that results from compression of the median nerve at the wrist. Current theory is that (1) the wear and tear of repetitive use causes the tendons to swell, pressing into the nerve in the tunnel, (2) bone dislocation or facture causes the bones to impinge upon the nerve, or (3) fluid retention causes swelling of tissue in the carpal tunnel. In addition, atmosphere in the workplace is seen to directly affect health with stress.

Transverse carpal ligament

Hamate   **Trapezium**

Symptoms of carpal tunnel syndrome include pain in the fingers, hands, forearms, shoulder and / or upper back. The pain can range from constant to occasional to burning or shooting pain to numbness to tingling. Loss of sensation and feeling or a "pins and needles" or "fall asleep" feeling are major signs of trouble. The net result of repetitive stress injury can be (1) a feeling of fatigue and weakness in the arms and hands, (2) dropping things and losing one's grip, (3) stiffness or difficulty in using one's hands, (4) hyperawareness or extreme sensitivity of the hands and fingers, and (5) chronically cold hands and frequent unconscious rubbing of one's hands and fingers.

Self-help exercises of directional movement of the hand are suggested for carpal tunnel syndrome. Frequent breaks away from the work station are suggested, in addition to use of an ergonomically correct work position. The stress of carpal tunnel syndrome includes stress in the neck, upper back, shoulders, and arm.

Trigger Finger

Trigger finger is the (1) snapping and clicking in the fingers when one bends or straightens the fingers (or thumb) or (2) the locking of the digit either fully bent or straightened. Normally the tendons that link muscle to bone and cause the fingers to bend pass through a tunnel that holds them attached to the finger bones. Trigger finger is an irritation of the digital sheath which surrounds the flexor tendons. When the tendon sheath becomes thickened or swollen, it pinches the tendon and prevents it from gliding smoothly. In some cases the tendon catches and then suddenly releases as though a "trigger" was released.

This condition usually occurs near the crease in the middle of the palm of the hand, and the patient feels pain in this area as well as over the top of the finger. Frequently, the clicking and locking becomes worse overnight, but as the patient uses the finger during the day, the symptoms improve.

Ganglion cysts

A ganglion cyst is a lump or bump commonly occurring at the back of the wrist or in the palm of the hand at the base of the finger. These non-cancerous, fluid-filled cysts arise from the ligaments, joint linings, or tendon sheaths when they are irritated or inflamed. They may disappear or change size quickly. They are more frequently seen in women, and the reason for their occurrence is unknown. One explanation is that they occur where there is a weak place in a joint capsule that develops a "blowout." This area forms a balloon-like extension of a joint with a one-way valve from the joint. Joint fluid can then flow into the balloon through the one-way flap valve but cannot return to the joint. Therefore, the ganglion cyst generally becomes larger and larger. Ganglion cysts can also be seen in and around tendons.

The relationship between ganglion cyst formation and physical exertion, occupation and injury is not totally understood. Since these are not cancerous lumps, one can feel comfortable leaving the cyst alone as long as it is not bothersome. Many years ago, doctors recommended hitting a ganglion with a large book (usually the Bible as it was the largest book available) and thus rupturing the sac. Many ganglion cysts do not require treatment.

Tendonitis of the Wrist

Tendonitis of the wrist is most common in adult women between the ages of 30 and 50. It is an irritation and swelling of the sheath or tunnel which surrounds the thumb tendons as they pass from the wrist to the thumb. Pain when grasping or pinching and tenderness over the tunnel are the most common symptoms. Sometimes a lump or thickening can be felt in this area. If the hand is made into a fist with the thumb "tucked in" and bent towards the little finger, the pain gets worse (Finkelstein test).

Tendonitis may be caused by overuse and also can be seen in association with pregnancy or inflammatory arthritis such as rheumatoid disease. If treated early, many cases improve with rest in a splint, injection with steroids and/or taking anti-inflammatory medications. More severe cases or those that do not respond to other treatment may require surgery. Modification of the activities which caused the symptoms initially also may be required.

Arthritis

Arthritis is a chronic inflammatory disease that primarily affects the joints and surrounding tissues. Rheumatoid arthritis is an autoimmune disease (your immune system attacks your own body). The immune system attacks the cells lining the joints (synovium). The linings of the joints become inflamed and it secretes more fluid than usual. The linings of the joints thicken. The disease process eventually erodes the cartilage, tendons and ligaments of the joint.

Thumb Arthritis

The thumb is generally considered to be the most important single digit in the hand. Working in opposition to the fingers it makes possible movements of the hands necessary for independent living such as buttoning, zipping, cooking and bathroom functions. This "wear and tear" arthritis is common.

The basal joint of the thumb, or carpometacarpal joint, is made up of a carpal or wrist bone (trapezium) and the first or metacarpal bone of the thumb. Arthritis is a common term meaning inflammation of a joint. Although arthritis can apply to more than 100 different diseases, the three most common types affecting the basal joint of the thumb are osteoarthritis (degenerative arthritis), rheumatoid arthritis, and traumatic arthritis (generally due to a fracture in the joint).

The basal joint of the thumb is subjected to an unusual amount of stress, as the thumb must be strong enough to counteract the force of four fingers put together. It has been calculated that one pound of pinch between the thumb and index finger will produce six-to-nine pounds of pressure at the basal joint of the thumb. The joint is held in position by the contours of its surface and by the ligaments and muscles surrounding the joint. Disruptions of the joint surface or the supporting ligaments can lead to slipping of the joint (subluxation) as well as pain and swelling.

Symptoms of arthritis in the base of the thumb are pain and swelling about the thumb and wrist, particularly with grasp and pinch. These symptoms may appear the first thing in the morning and be present for a half hour or so before the thumb "loosens up." They might then subside throughout the middle of the day, only to return with a "dull aching" type of pain towards the end of the day or after vigorous use. A "bump" may appear at the joint, due to the shifting of the base of the metacarpal bone as the ligaments loosen through swelling.

Heberden nodes

Heberden nodes are "bumps" which occur at the last joint of the finger or thumb due to wear and tear arthritis (osteoarthritis). As the joints deteriorate, small bone spurs form over the back of the joints and make them appear "lumpy." Individuals should continue moving their hands; disuse frequently results in stiffness.

Circulatory Dysfunctions

Circulatory functioning of the blood of the hand may be impacted by high blood pressure /hypertension, hypothyroidism (a deficiency of thyroid activity), obesity, or acute renal failure. A sudden decline in renal function may be triggered by a number of acute disease processes. Examples include sepsis (infection), shock, trauma, kidney stones, kidney infection, drug toxicity (aspirin or lithium), poisons or toxins (drug abuse) or after injection with an iodinated contrast dye (adverse effect).

Nervous system dysfunctions

Nerve circulation in the hand may be impacted by diabetes.

Appearance of the Nails

Appearance of the Nails as an Indicator of Disease

Fingernails are often are a key indicator of disease far from the hands. These include diabetes, liver disease and kidney disease and this is why physicians always scan your hands during an examination. The fingernails are viewed as a window into health - their thin transparent appearance provides a glance into the blood vessels which flow under them. Thus, the appearance of the fingernails mirrors the color of the blood.

• All-white nails may indicate liver problems, while those half-pink and half white may point to kidney disorders.

• Signs of diabetes include a yellowish tint and a slight pink coloring at the base of the nail.

• Yellow color can indicate lung illness (tuberculosis, asthma and fungal infections).

• Whitish color may be indicative of chronic hepatisis or cirrhosis.

• A pale color may mean anemia.

• Bluish nails may be a sign of circulation problem. A bluish color has been connected to chronic lung disorder such as emphysema or asthma. It may mean heart failure and exposure to toxins such as copper or silver.

• Excess of iron could turn the nails gray, blue or brown in color.

• If a nail is half and half (half normal color, half white horizontally) it may be the result of kidney disorders.

• Horizontal white lines can result from chemotherapy which may slow or stop nail growth during treatment. This is usually a brief reaction. They could be a reaction to drugs while the nails were forming. They may follow an infectious disease or could reflect recent surgery.

• Black, splinterlike small areas under the nails are actually small hemorrhages and may indicate infection of the heart valves. They may also be an indicator of lupus or trichinosis.

Color isn't the only indicator of the relationship between health and fingernails.

• Brittle nails may indicate dehydration especially if they split.

• Breaking-splitting fingernails could be a sign of thyroid problems.

• Misshapen nails maybe a sign of arthritis or nutritional

deficiency.

• Extremely rounded or clubbed nails may indicate congenital heart disease, lung cancer, or other chronic heart or lung conditions such as tuberculosis.
• Some things are harmless, such as little white spots, which can result from low grade infections.

Nail Disorders and Other Influences on the Fingernail Appearance

Nails can have their own problems. Dermatologists report common nail problems are infections from bacteria, such as staphylococcus; fungi, such as Candida (also known as yeast); and skin viruses, such as warts.
Nutrition can effect the nails. Fingernails require complete protein and calcium. Vitamins A, C and B Complex, and other minerals such as sulfur and iodine are important for healthy nails. Iron is necessary to prevent weak, dry, thin nails. Vitamin C serves to prevent peeling and hangnails and B Complex prevents fragile nails.

Some harm can be self inflicted. Bacterial and fungal infections frequently result from artificial nails, whether applied at home or in a salon. Nail beds can be damaged by improper application of artificial nails when gaps are formed and bacterial agents invade.

The Body's Stress Mechanism

The goal of this section is twofold (1) to note how stress impacts the body and its parts and (2) to present a physiological explanation of how reflexology works within the nervous system.

Stress Mechanism: Tone in the Autonomic Nervous System

Tone is the body's basic internal communication system. It is the background against which the events of the day are played. We most often think of tone in terms of weight lifters and muscle development. Muscle tone provides the continuity to move the body through the day and to serve as a starting point to carry out various activities. Tone also exists in the internal organs and serves the same purpose of providing both a starting point and a means of continuity as the body attempts to meet the demands of the day. It is in this way that the body maintains and communicates every ongoing process. It is a priority system which maintains the internal organization in spite of rapid changes in the external environment.

Tone in the body's internal environment is maintained by the autonomic nervous system (hereafter referred to as ANS). The ANS is a part of the nervous system which regulates bodily functions which are beyond conscious control. It works by way of reflex action, adjusting a wide variety of balances. The ANS governs functions such as heart beat, the secretion of digestive juices and the ventilation of the body's heating system. These functions occur without conscious monitoring, but they require the gathering of information from the entire body. This calls for a synchronized system which can meet the demands of an emergency as well as normal day to day activities. Once the decision is made to fight, flee or make peace in reaction to a situation, the ANS is the physiological means by which the body carries out the decision in reference to the internal organs.

The ANS has two divisions to meet the variety of demands placed upon it. The sympathetic division (**II**) is the action mode of operation, the doer. While it is concerned with degrees of "fight or flight" responses to stimuli, it is not simply reserved for emergencies. It is called upon when there is a need for the activities of movement, of thinking, and of certain emotions.

II

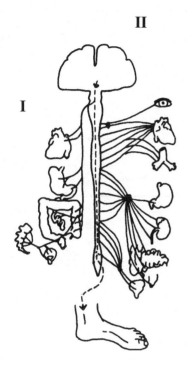

I

The parasympathetic division (**I**) is a conservor. It is concerned with vegetative functions such ʿ secretory activity and peristalsis. In paraplegia, for example, when voluntary movement of major parts of the body is limited or impossible, the internal organs are maintained by the parasympathetic division.

There is a complex interaction between the two divisions. Basically, the interaction is one of excitation of an organ by one division and inhibition of the activities by the other division. Tone is the balance which exists between the two to ensure smooth operations. This balance is the result of hereditary factors and a lifetime of learning. Just as with any learning situation, the more time a body spends practicing" or just being in sympathetic mode, for example, the more proficient it becomes at it. The parasympathetic mode must adjust to the sympathetic level, in this example.

Problems occur when the relationship between the two divisions becomes inflexible. An analogy from the mechanical world is the grinding and eventual wearing down of the starter in a car. Repeated, regular demands on the starter, especially after the engine is running, cause wear and eventual failure. Constant sympathetic demands, for example, such as the constant anxiety and repressed anger reported in high blood pressure patients, eventually wears on the appropriate body part. The complexity of the ANS provides almost limitless combinations of wear on the body. Since the ANS innervates every internal organ, a lack of flexibility in the balance in the ANS can affect any organ in the body.

Sensory input, whether it be in the form of sight or information on the terrain underfoot, makes complex demands on the body. The ANS is the means by which the internal organs respond to these demands. A repetitious sameness in sensory experience offers a sameness of demand on and response by the body, resulting in an inflexibility in the system. Reflexology is one means of varying sensory experience and, thus, encouraging flexibility in the internal environment.

How Does Reflexology Work? Reflex Conditioning

"reflex;... Esp. Physiol. designating or of an involuntary action as a sneeze resulting when a stimulus is carried by an afferent (sensory) nerve to a nerve center and the response is reflected along an afferent (motor) nerve to some muscle or gland." (*Webster's Third World Dictionary*, New York, Simon & Schuster, p. 1193)

Pressure sensors in the hands are a part of the body's reflexive network that makes possible a fight or flight response. In case of danger, the hands reach for a weapon, the feet prepare to fight or flee, and the internal organs provide adrenaline, oxygen, and glucose to fuel the effort. On a more mundane level, this same mechanism propels us through the day, taking us to work and moving us about our activities.

Many of the hand's activities are learned in childhood, but the learning never actually stops. We constantly receive feedback from the environment about where we are and what we are doing. The perception of pressure by the hand provides feedback about what is in hand. Such demands create a need for a response appropriate to the occasion.

Every day is not a new day for the hand or any other sensory organ. Using information gathered over a lifetime, instructions for sensory organs are preprogrammed in anticipation of events to come. The responses to our environment are preset programs of muscular tension fed forward to appropriate body parts from the brain. In other words, to continually respond to our changing environment, we need to receive feedback from our senses and to respond with "feed forward" directions from our brain. The classic example of a sensory organ receiving feed forward instructions occurs when a mother hears her infant cry. A mother can differentiate her own infant's crying from other infants because her hearing mechanism is tuned to her baby's cry. Thus specific instructions about that baby's cry are provided or fed forward by the brain.

It is this feed back / feed forward loop for sensory organs that makes possible a reflexology influence on the whole body. At the same time that a sensory organ such as the hand is being sent instructions from the brain, the internal organs are also receiving instructions. These instructions are about the levels of oxygen and fuel necessary to make movement possible. Although many parts of the brain are involved in this process, there is one final, common pathway in the brain stem that sends instructions to both the hands and the internal organs. The manipulating mechanism of the hand is, thus, linked to the internal organs.

Any pressure perceived by the hand is a stimulus to which the entire body responds. Changes throughout the nervous system result from the perception of pressure by the hand. A discussion follows about the physiology of a pressure reflex and its role in the conditioning of the body.

Conditioning the Nervous System

"A conversation at a cocktail party will change your life," said Sir Charles Sherrington, neurologist and Nobel prize winner. It was not the content of the conversation to which he referred. It was the physical impingement of a voice on a nervous system that he considered. Sherrington was actually noting that, by definition, any sensory input changes the nervous system that perceives it.

A sensation of pressure from the hand travels from the skin inward along the route of the nervous system causing the body to adjust in a number of ways. Over time, continued exposure to pressure will cause these adjustments to be a more permanent fixture of the nervous system. The learning and conditioning that take place create a change in homeostasis or what the Russians referred to as brain-organ dynamics. The body, thus, alters its behavior and learns to act in the best manner possible.

From the Selye model, stress is a part of life. With only so much energy available to respond to stress, the best possible adaptation to stress is one that results in the least wear and tear on the body. New sensory input provides a break in the continuity of the established stress pattern. An interruption of the stress lessens its impact.

Conditioning Change in the Nervous System

Conditioning change in the nervous system is possible because the hand plays an integral role in the survival function. Patterns to cope with the stress of locomotion are formed in the hand itself, between body parts, and throughout the body as a whole. Those patterns of stress are:

Hand Stress: An overall tension level in the hand is necessary to maintain a readiness to manipulate.

Reflex Stress: An overall tension level between body parts is necessary to integrate movement and the fuel needed to move.

Body Stress: A background level of tension is necessary to provide a continuous response to the internal and external environments.

The hand requires energy to make its contribution to movement. Too much energy expended in locomotion results in wear and tear throughout the body. The application of pressure techniques to the hand interrupts stress and creates the following changes in the nervous system:

Tension: Change in the overall body tone or stress level to create relaxation.

Body Image: Alteration of the body's picture of itself to create a more accurate perception.

Metabolic Rate: Changes in metabolism to create a more efficient response to stress.

Homeostasis, Brain / Organ Dynamics / Autonomic Regulation: By any name, changes in the overall operating balance of the body.

The entire body adjusts in response to demands such as the stress of a pressure sensation. Each pressure sensory input alters the reflex image, the body image that is shared by all body parts. Adjustment is provided in the dynamic state of tension maintained to produce the best possible condition for the body and its functions. Reflexology utilizes pressure applied to a significant part of the body to interrupt stress and to create a break in routine that helps resolve the wear-and-tear aspect of stress.

Autonomic Nervous System and Central Nervous System

In case of danger, the brain communicates with the internal organs through the autonomic nervous system and the muscles, such as those of the hand, through the central nervous system. The reflexive response to a pressure stimulus also requires a response by the autonomic nervous system and the central nervous system.

Sensory information flows to the brain and, after being evaluated flows back to every part of the body that requires this information. Now the brain "feeds forward" two sets of instructions. One set of instructions is for the readiness of the internal organs. The other set of instructions is for the level of muscular tension. For these purposes, detailed instructions project an image of the body back down the spinal cord and through cranial nerves to the entire nervous system. Instructions to the autonomic portion of the nervous system are relayed to the parasympathetic portion by way of the cranial nerves emanating from the brain stem. Instructions to the sympathetic portion of the autonomic nervous system are projected through the reticular core, down the spinal cord to thoracic and lumbar nerves they activate.

Instructions to the locomotor apparatus, such as the hand, (1) change existing background tone in pressure, stretch, and movement (proprioceptive) sensors and (2) create movement. Thus, the reflexive action created in response to a pressure sensation includes new instructions to the pressure sensor where the reflexive activity originated. Not only will the pressure sensor be changed by pressure, but the whole body will also feel the influence.

CHAPTER 5

Pressure Techniques

Pressure is a sensation that is felt by the hands. Pressure sensors in the hand make possible the manipulation of our world. Both the fine stroke of a pen and the lifting of a weight call for pressure sensitivity. In reflexology, the goal is the application of constant steady pressure to all parts of the hand. To reach this goal in this chapter, we will consider the specific techniques for the working and holding hands.

During technique application, control is an important element. Control is the ability to most efficiently and effectively apply techniques. The net result of steady control is a sense of precision, comfort, confidence and thoroughness. Control is achieved by placement of the client's hand on a padded surface and the interplay of the practitioner's two hands. Throughout the Technique chapter, techniques are described in terms of two steps: the preparation made by a holding hand and the application of technique made by a working hand. Further references to the terms 'working hand' and 'holding hand' describe the practitioner's role. Any reference to "the hand" can be interpreted as the hand being worked.

The goal of the reflexologist is to most efficiently and effectively combine the efforts of the working hand and holding hand. Toward this purpose, the role of the practitioner's hands is to steady the hand being worked and to apply a sensory signal to the hand being worked.

The technique illustrations show the position off the holding hand and the working hand. To work with the illustrations, make it a practice to note and then mimic the roles played by each hand. The holding hand creates a stationary target and appropriate conditions for the working hand, The working hand applies techniques that create the sensation of pressure.

To consider the role of the holding hand, rest your hands on a table with the palmar surface up. Note that the fingers curl and the thumb draws toward the hand. A hand being worked will display this natural tendency. To create a more appropriate condition for the working hand, the holding hand comes into play, easing the fingers and thumb into a stretched position thus creating a flattened, less fleshy working surface.

To consider the role of the working hand, look at the palm of your hand. Note that the contours of the hand provide a variety of surface. The thumb, fingers, joints, webbings, and palm of the hand provide distinctively different surfaces that the working hand must accommodate.

Thumb Walking Technique

The goal of thumb walking technique is to exert a constant steady pressure while contouring to the surface of the hands.

The interplay of the fingers and thumb provide the ability to contour and exert pressure to a variety of surfaces. The fingers act in unison to grasp, while the thumb is free to provide pressure in opposition is a very precise manner. The tip of the thumb is the point of contact for the exertion of pressure. The natural angle of the thumb is such that the outside edge works optimally in opposition to the fingers to create pressure.

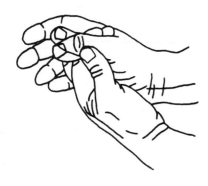

The thumb walking technique has a very simple basis: the bending of the first joint of the thumb. Try this exercise: hold the thumb below the first joint (as shown). This prevents the second joint form bending. Bend the first joint. Do it several times. Now try the other thumb.

While you're still holding, place the outside corner of the thumb on your leg. Bend the thumb a few times. At this point, do not worry about exerting pressure or about what your other fingers are doing.

The next step is to get your thumb actually walking forward. Hold on to your thumb. Use the outside tip. Bend

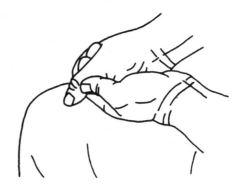

the thumb, allowing it to rock a little form the thumb tip to the lower edge of the thumbnail. This is not a large range of motion; it is not meant to be.

Remove the holding had. Try walking the thumb. Are you bending only the first joint? Do not push the thumb forward. Bending and unbending is the entire means by which you move forward.

It is at this point that an important aspect of efficiency arises. The fact is that actual strength in reflexology comes form the use of the four fingers in opposition to the thumb.

To practice the thumb walking technique, first imagine trying to grasp a chin-up bar. The hands are in an open grasp, with the fingers holding on. Think in terms of a three-stage process.

Grasp: Grasp the arm.

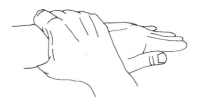

Lift off: unwrap the thumb form the grasp. Maintain the grasp of the fingers.

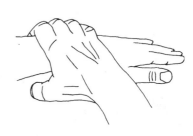

Contact: Place the tip of the thumb on the surface of the arm. The outside edge is the point of contact. The finger-tips maintain the grasp. The hand arcs between the fingertips and the edge of the thumb. A downward pressure by the thumb tip is thus created. The pressure varies with the tension created between the thumb and fingers. An increase of pull by the finger, by lowering the wrist, increases the pressure exerted by the thumb tip.

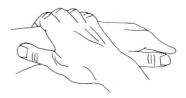

With the thumb tip on the surface of the arm and the thumb held straight, drop the wrist. Note the increased pressure by the thumb tip.

The object of thumb walking technique is to exert a constant, steady pressure with the thumb tip. The entire hand participates in this technique, but the first joint of the thumb is the only moving part. The first joint bends and unbends to move the thumb tip in a forward direction. The second joint of the thumb does not move. It participates in the creation of leverage and, thus, pressure.

The Roles of the Holding Hand and the Working Hand

In applying the thumb walking technique to the hand, the roles of the holding hand and the working hand are considered. The holding hand positions the hand being worked to prepare a more suitable surface on which to work, one which is stationary and held taut to thin the flesh. The working hand provides the sensory signal of pressure. Pressure is exerted at the thumb tip, but the entire hand participates in the exertion of pressure and contouring to the surface being worked.

To practice the thumb walking technique on the hand and to become familiar with the handling of the hand, work through the following exercises, applying the thumb walking technique after the hands have been positioned as indicated. In the thumb walking technique, the thumb moves in a forward direction. Note that the working hand is positioned to allow the thumb to move forward and to contour to the surface.

Applied Techniques

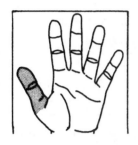 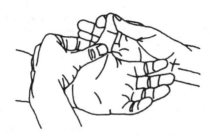

Holding hand (R): Hold the thumb stationary.
Working hand (L): Fingers rest on top side of hand to provide leverage by opposing the thumb

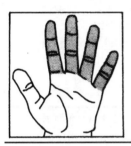 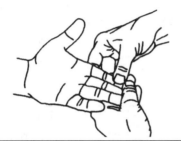

Holding hand (L): Grasp the fingers to prevent them from curling.
Working hand (R): Fingers rest on top side of hand.

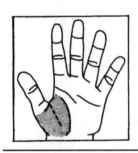 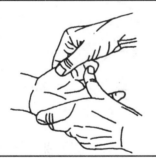

Holding hand (L): Thr thumb is braced and drawn away from the hand.
Working hand (R): Fingers rest on top side of hand. The four fingers rest together to best create leverage.

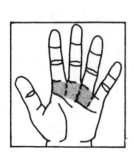 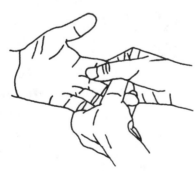

Holding hand (L): Grasp the fingers to open the palm of the hand.
Working hand (R): Fingers rest on top side of hand. Note the intended direction of the working thumb.

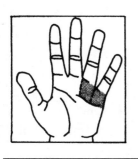 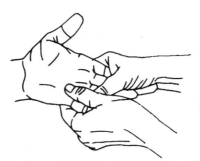

Holding hand (R): Grasp the fingers to open the palm of the hand.
Working hand (L): Fingers rest together on the top side of the hand.

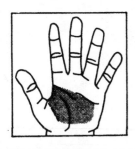 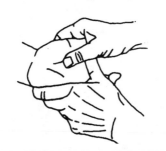

Holding hand (R): The thumb is drawn away from the body of the hand to more fully expose the webbing of the hand.
Working hand (L): Fingers rest on the top side of the hand.

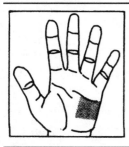 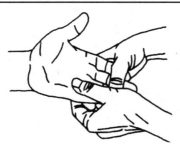

Holding hand (R): Grasp the fingers to open the palm of the hand.
Working hand (L): Fingers rest on the top side of the hand. The left hand is used to more easily work toward the outside of the palm.

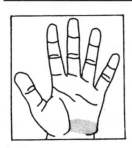 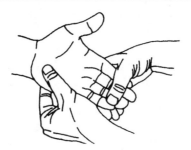

Holding hand (R): Grasp the fingers to open the palm of the hand.
Working hand (L): As compared to the previous picture, the working hand has been repositioned. The working hand is repositioned to allow the working thumb to move within a comfortable range. Loss of leverage occurs when the thumb is stretched beyond the range of comfort.

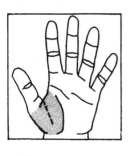 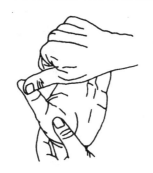

Holding hand (R): Use the palm to hold the fingers and open the palm of the hand. The thumb is braced and spread away from the body of the hand.

Working hand (L): Fingers rest together on the top side of the hand. Note the intended direction of the working thumb.

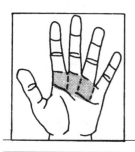 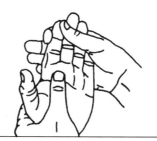

Holding hand (R): Grasp the fingers, using the thumb to stretch the fingers, to open the palm of the hand and create a less fleshy surface for the working hand.

Working hand (L): Fingers rest on the top side of the hand.

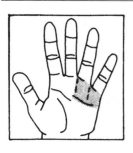 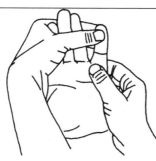

Holding hand (R): Grasp the finger to open the palm of the hand and use the fingertips of the holding hand to spread the fingers to more easily allow technique application into the webbing.

Working hand (L): Begin thumb walking technique passes at, the base of the metacarpal head.

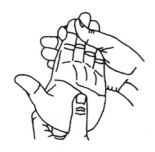

Complete the coverage of the palmar surface. Determine which hand most easily contours to the surface and is the most appropriate working hand.

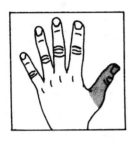 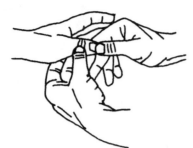

Holding hand (R): Hold the thumb to steady it.

Working hand (L): Rest the fingers on the palm side of the thumb to provide leverage.

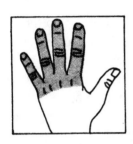 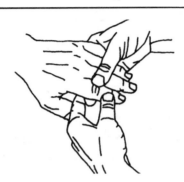

Holding hand (R): Hold the finger to steady it. For comfort and control, all four fingers are grasped with the fingertips of the working hand positioning the finger.

Working hand (L): Rest the fingers on the palmar surface.

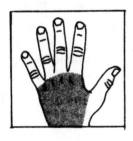 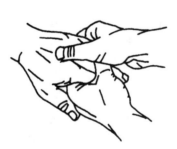

Holding hand (R): Grasp the fingers to steady the hand.

Working hand (L): Note that the right hand most easily works toward the outside of the hand.

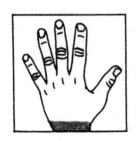 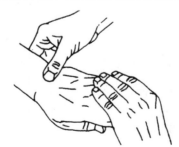

Holding hand (R): Grasp the fingers to steady the hand.

Working hand (L): Note the intended direction of the working thumb

Finger Walking Technique

The finger walking technique has the same basis as the thumb walking technique: the bending of the first joint of the finger. Hold the finger below the first joint (as shown). Bend the first joint.

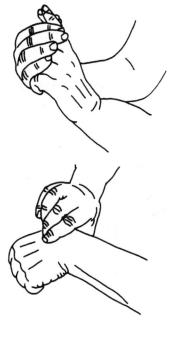

The top of the hand is a good practice ground for finger walking. Try bending from the first joint of the index finger as its tip rests on top of the hand. Use the edge of the finger. The walking motion is a slight rocking from the fingertip to the lower edge of the fingernail.

To apply the finger walking technique to the hand, note that the finger contours to the top side of the hand. Note the positions of the working hand and holding hand. The thumb of the working hand is positioned on the palm side of the hand and it provides leverage for the working finger. The finger walks in a forward direction. The starting point establishes the direction of the walking finger.

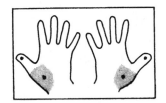

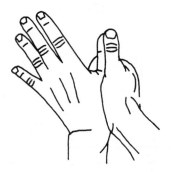

Modified Hook and Back Up Technique

The modified hook and back up technique is used to pin-point in the fleshier portions of the hand. The possibility of contact between the fingernail of the working finger and the hand is a consideration in the application of technique. An effort should be made not to make contact between the fingernail and the hand.

To practice the technique on yourself, grasp the hand as shown. The palm of the working hand rests on the top side of the hand. The tip of the finger is placed on the area to be worked. The palm acts with a bracing effect and the tip of the finger makes contact to exert pressure. Exert pressure with the fingertip. Note your own reaction to the fingernail contact. When working on another's hand, fingernail contact is to be avoided. To avoid contact, the flat of the finger exerts the pressure.

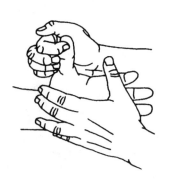

To apply the modified hook and back up technique to the hand, rest the palm of the working hand on the top side of the hand. Note the position of the holding hand to control the hand when technique is applied to the thumb and create a smooth working surface when technique is applied to the thenar eminence. Place the fingertip on the area to be worked. Exert pressure repeatedly with the flat of the finger

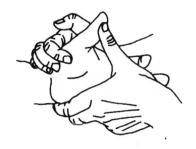

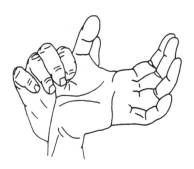

Rotating on a Point

The rotating on a point technique is used to pinpoint in the bonier portions of the hand.

The working hand grasps the wrist, pinpointing with the flat of the finger. The holding hand moves the hand first in a clockwise and then in a counterclockwise direction.

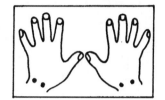 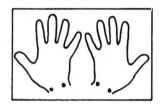

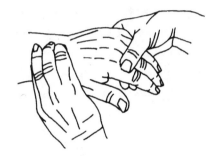 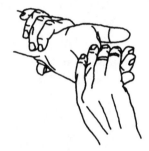

Variation

The va....on is an aggressive technique and not for application to everyone. Apply carefully. The hand is held in an upright position. The working hand grasps the wrist, pinpointing with the flat of the thumb. Note the position of the working thumb. The holding hand moves the hand first in a clockwise direction for several circles and then in a counterclockwise direction.

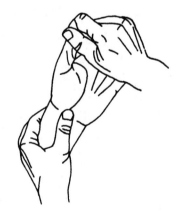

69

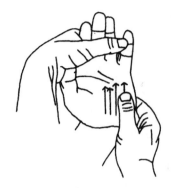

Establishing a Pattern of Successive Passes

In applying the thumb walking technique to the hand, a pattern of successive passes is established. Such a pattern provides pathways for the walking thumb and a thorough coverage of the surface of the hand. A series of passes is applied to cover a segment of the hand surface. The hand is held in position while successive passes of the thumb walking technique are made (See illustration.) The position of the holding hand is then changed and a new series of successive passes is applied. The net result is an effective, efficient, and thorough application of pressure to the hand.

To practice successive passes of the thumb walking technique on the hand, work through the following exercise. The placement of the thumb to begin a pass establishes the pathway for the thumb walking technique. The thumb always moves in a forward direction.

Note the changing position of the working hand to accommodate placement of the thumb for the next pass. Note the positions of the working hand and holding hand. Note the starting position for the working thumb. To make a pass, walk the thumb in a forward direction. The pass ends when the thumb is stretched beyond the ability to take advantage of the leverage provided by the fingers. To begin another pass, reposition the thumb.

Note the placement of the working hand and holding hand. Note the position of the four fingers of the working hand which provide opposition to the thumb, thus creating leverage and controlling the pressure applied by the walking thumb. Begin a series of thumb walking passes.

In the following exercises, establish pathways and create successive passes of the thumb walking technique. Take note of:
• The starting position of the working thumb
• The positions of the working hand and the holding hand
• The position of the working finger.

Visualize the segment of the hand to be covered. Begin a series of successive passes, thoroughly and repeatedly covering the segment.

Thenar eminence: Hand held horizontally

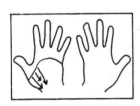
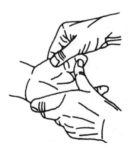
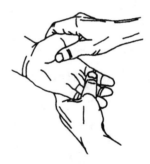

Thenar eminence: Hand held vertically

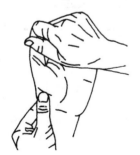
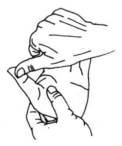
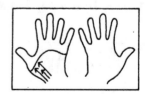

Ball of the hand: Hand held horizontally

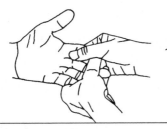 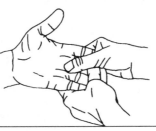 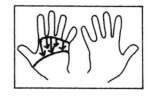

Ball of the hand: Hand held vertically

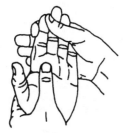 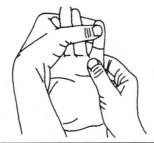 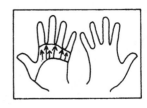

Body of the hand: Hand held horizontally

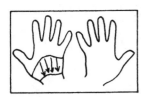 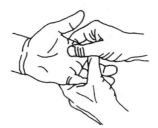 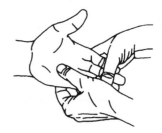

Body of the hand: Hand held vertically

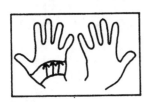 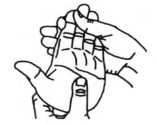 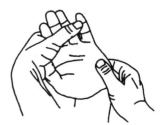

Top of the hand

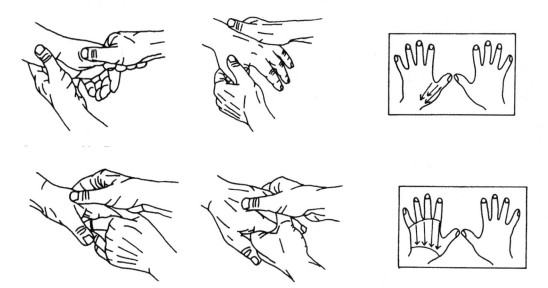

CHAPTER 6

Technique Application Appropriate to Each Reflex Area

The techniques described in this book are designed to achieve two main goals: efficiency and effectiveness in applying pressure technique to the hands. In reflexology, efficiency is covering a reflex area with the least amount of effort. Effectiveness is hitting the point, being dead-on-the-target in every reflex area. This chapter provides an exercise in applying successive passes while locating each reflex area.

Palmar Surface

The Thumb

pituitary

thyroid / parathyroid

seventh cervical

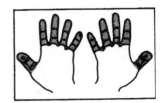

The thumb includes several important reflex areas. Each

thumb represents half of the head reflex area and contains all five zones. The head joins onto the body just as the thumb joins the hand. The important connector between the thumb and the hand then corresponds to the neck.

The **pituitary** is an exact pinpoint reflex area. The pituitary reflex area lies in the center of the first segment of the thumb.

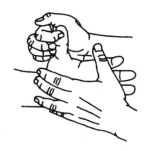

To work the point, support and protect the thumb with the palm of the working hand. The holding hand spreads the finger and opens up the palm to more clearly expose the thumb. Place the working finger just beyond the pituitary reflex area. Apply the modified *hook and back up* technique several times.

The **thyroid/parathyroid** reflex areas are located in the proximal phalanx of the thumb and fingers. For the moment, we will discuss the technique for working this reflex area on the thumb.

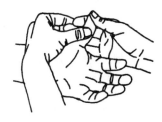

To work the thyroid/parathyroid reflex area, support and protect the thumb with the holding hand. Use the holding thumb to hold the thumb and to provide a stationary target. Place the fingers of the working hand on those of the holding hand. Walk across the area using the *thumb walking* technique. Make at least two passes, one high and one low. Several passes are necessary in order to cover the thyroid's wide reflex area. By working this and the seventh cervical reflex area, you will have covered the entire base of the thumb.

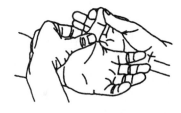

The **seventh cervical** affects everything from the neck to the fingertips. Numbness in the fingers can often be traced to the seventh cervical. To work the seventh cervical, start by anchoring the thumb with the fingertips and thumb. Place the working fingers in a comfortable position on the top of the hand. Walk forward with the thumb around the base of the thumb.

The Fingers: Thumb Walking

head / brain / sinuses

jaw / teeth / gums

neck / thyroid / throat

The fingers represent a breakdown of the thumb. They are in zones 2, 3, 4, and 5, respectively. The goal of this technique is to walk the thumb around the padded surfaces and joints of the fingers.

Begin by supporting and holding in place the fingers with the holding hand in a horizontal position. The fingers curl naturally and would be difficult to work if not stretched flat. Place the fingers of the working hand on the holding fingers. Walk with the thumb across the finger.

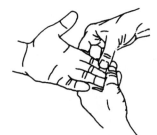 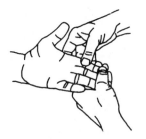 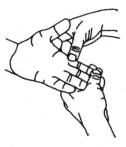

Now hold the hand upright vertically. (Not illustrated.) The fingers of the holding hand rest on the dorsal surface of the hand, stretching and holding the fingers in place. The thumb and finger tips of the holding hand hold the finger being worked. Starting at the base of the index finger, walk with the thumb. Go on to work the other fingers in a similar manner, moving the fingers of the holding hand to support and hold the finger being worked.

The interphalangeal joint at the base of the middle phalanx represents the jaw / teeth reflex area. The padded area of the proximal phalanx represents the neck / thyroid / parathyroid reflex area. The padded area of the distal phalanx represents the head/brain area.

Ball of the Hand

eye / ear / tops of shoulders

chest/lung/breast

shoulder

solar plexus / diaphragm

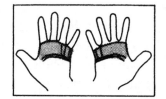

The object of this technique is to walk with the thumb along the heads of the metacarpal bones. To maximize effectiveness, the flesh in this area must be thinned out.

Hold the hand horizontally. With the holding hand, pull the fingers back to thin out this flesh (as shown). This opens the area. The fingers of the working hand rest on the dorsal surface of the hand. Begin thumb walking technique passes at the medial side of the first metacarpal head. Contour the moving thumb to the medial side in one pass, to the center of the metacarpal head in another pass, and the lateral side of the metacarpal heads. Move on to the other metacarpal heads successively.

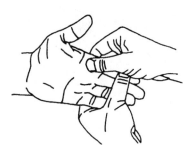

Technique application to the hand held horizontally works through the lung/chest/breast area with the pass ending in the solar plexus/diaphragm reflex area. The fifth metacarpal represents the shoulder reflex area.

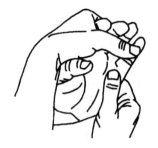

Now hold the hand vertically. Place the thumb of the right hand at the base of the fifth metacarpal head, the solar plexus / diaphragm reflex area. The left hand acts as the holding hand, supporting the hand and stretching the fingers flat. Make a series of successive passes, contouring the working thumb to the medial side of the metacarpal head, the center and then the lateral side.

As you apply technique between the metacarpal heads, move into the webbing between the second and third fingers. Make several passes in this small area, simultaneously using thumb and finger walking techniques. Notice that the working index finger serves as a backstop for the working thumb. Make several passes through the webbing. The reflex area represented is that of the eyes and tops of shoulders.

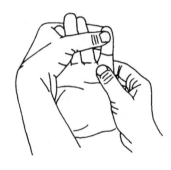

Move on to work with the fourth metacarpal head and webbing between the third and fourth fingers.

To work with the metacarpal head of the second and third digits, change working and holding hands so that the left hand becomes the working hand the right hand the holding hand. The working hand more easily reaches the surface to the medial side of the hand. Make a series of successive passes, contouring the working thumb to the medial side of the third metacarpal head, the center and then the lateral side. Make several passes through the webbing between the second and third fingers with the working thumb. Move on to the second metacarpal head.

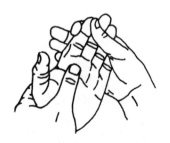

The fifth metacarpal head represents the shoulder reflex area. The webbing between the third and fourth finger represents the inner ear. The webbing between the fourth and fifth fingers represents the ear reflex area.

Note: In general, the hand follows a logical pattern relating the anatomy of the body to reflex areas on the hand. The location of the eye/ear reflex area seems to be an exception. Even though the reflexes of the eyes and ears are probably located in the fingers themselves, this part of the hand represents the muscles on the tops of the shoulders, which support the head and neck. The cranial nerves that provide innervation to the eyes and ears emerge from under the skull into the neck muscles.

Thenar Eminence and Webbing: Thumb Walking

adrenal gland

stomach

pancreas

kidney

upper back

scapula (collar bone)

ribs

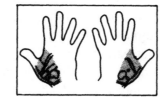

As you can see from the list above, many vital organs are represented in the thenar eminence and webbing of the hand. The thumb walking technique is used to work all of these reflexes in a systematic way. For maximum effectiveness it is necessary to be conscious of the specific organ's reflex location.

The region is bounded by the diaphragm and the waist-line. (See Illus.) On the hand, the diaphragm reflex area is defined by the metacarpophalangeal joint of the thumb. The waistline is an imaginary line drawn across the hand at the bases of the metacarpal bones. Find this bone on your own hand. Then draw a line from the high spot on this bone straight across the hand. This is your waistline. As you can see, the waistline marker creates a much larger area above the waistline and a much smaller area below the waistline on the hand as opposed to the foot.

Another locator is the webbing of the hand between first and second metacarpal bones. The kidney reflex area lies to the lateral side of the webbing and into the deep part of the webbing formed between the first and second metacarpal bones. The adrenal gland reflex area lies midway down the first metacarpal bone and to the lateral side, bordering on the webbing. The pancreas reflex area lies along the midline of the first metacarpal bone.The stomach reflex area lies across the base of the first metacarpal bone. The majority of the pancreas reflex area is on the left hand. The webbing of the hand includes upper back, scapula, and rib reflex areas.

To apply technique to the deeply-seated adrenal reflex area, apply the modified hook and back up technique. Holding the left hand horizontally and using the right hand as a working hand, curl the index finger around the first metacarpal bone so that the tip of the index finger rests on the site for the adrenal reflex area. Exert pressure with the index fingers making several contacts.

To work the thenar eminence, hold the hand horizontally, palmar surface up. The right hand most easily serves as the working hand with the left hand. To try this

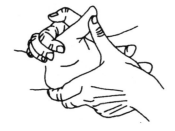

technique, stretch the fingers back with the holding hand. Use the holding thumb to place the thumb in a stretched position and flatten the fleshy working surface. Place the working thumb at the base of the thumb. Use the thumb walking technique to make several passes through the area.

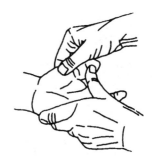

The webbing of the hand between the index finger and thumb provides a special working area. With the left hand held horizontally and the palmar surface up, use the left hand as a holding hand. Spread the thumb and fingers apart using the holding hand to hold the thumb and the fingers to hold the fingers. Rest the thumb tip of the working hand on the palmar surface of the webbing and index finger tip of the working hand on the dorsal surface. Use both thumb and finger walking simultaneously to work a pass through the webbing. The thumb and finger serve as a back stop against which each exerts pressure. Make several passes to cover the whole area.

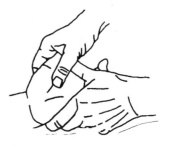

Technique may also be applied to this area by holding the hand vertically. To work with the left hand, use the right hand to hold the thumb and fingers in a stretched position. Use both thumb and finger walking simultaneously to work through the webbing.

The webbing represents musculo-skeletal reflex areas for the upper back, as well and scapula (collar bone) and ribs as well as several organs.

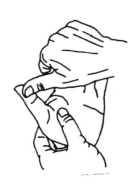

To apply technique to the thenar eminence with the hand held vertically, the holding hand stretches the fingers back and the holding thumb positions the thumb. Place the working thumb at the base of the first metacarpal bone. Use the thumb walking technique to make several passes through the area.

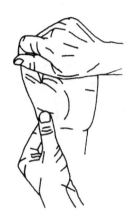

Body of the Hand:
Solar Plexus and Below

solar plexus / diaphragm

stomach (part)

pancreas (part)

liver and gallbladder / spleen

arm / elbow

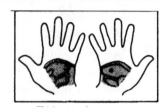

Hold the hand horizontally with the palmar surface up. On the left hand, the right hand most easily serves as the working hand to the medial areas of the body of the hand. The left hand most easily applies technique to the lateral areas. To try this technique on the left hand, use the left holding hand to stretch the fingers back. The flat of the working thumb rests on the second metacarpal head. With the thumb walking technique, make several passes throughout the area.

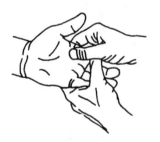

Change working and holding hands. Make several passes through the body of the hand in the area of the fourth and fifth metacarpal bones.
Hold the hand vertically. Proceed as with described above for the hand held horizontally.

Change working and holding hands. Make several passes throughout the body of the hand in the area of the fourth and fifth metacarpal bones.

The liver/gallbladder is a rather large reflex area under the diaphragm line. It extends from the outside of the right hand all the way across to the left hand. The gallbladder is located on the right hand, but may vary a bit in location.

The spleen is positioned under the diaphragm line on the left hand. Much smaller than the liver, it is located at the tail end of the pancreas.

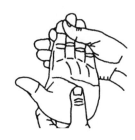

The stomach lies mostly on the left hand, overlapping several reflex areas. The duodenum, the prime candidate for ulceration, lies on the right hand, just to the outside edge of the pancreas.

Slightly above the waistline on both hands are parts of the large colon. Parts of the large intestine run through this reflex area. Working the large intestine, however, is discussed in the section on the waistline and below.

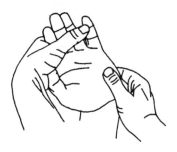

Body of the Hand Below the Waistline

Right Hand / Left Hand

colon / colon

ileocecal valve / sigmoid colon

small intestine / small intestine

kidney / kidney

lower back/hip/pelvis / lower back/hip/pelvis

Look at the heel of the right hand. Try to visualize the intestines superimposed on it. The transverse colon runs along a line formed by the base of the metacarpals. Starting at the fifth metatarsal, the ascending colon runs to the lateral side of the heel. On the right hand this reflex area includes half of the small intestine framed by the colon, and the ileocecal valve.

The ileocecal valve, which is located at the beginning of the colon, is worked by *pinpointing*. To find the ileocecal valve reflex point, run your hand down the outside of the hand into the heel. Hook into this spot and back across it with your index finger. The thumb provides the leverage.

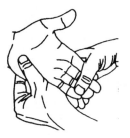

To work the heel of the left hand, hold the hand horizontally with the right holding hand. With the right holding hand, grasp the fingers and stretch the palm open. Rest the flat of the left working thumb on the surface of the heel of the hand and make several passes throughout the area. The sigmoid colon reflex area lies between the heel of the hand and the thenar eminence.

Hold the left hand vertically with the right holding hand, controlling the fingers and stretching the palm open. With the left working thumb make several successive passes through the area

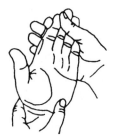

Wrist

ovary / testicle

uterus / prostate

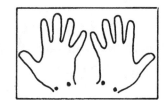

With the working hand, grasp the wrist pinpointing the ovary/testicle reflex area in the bony region of the wrist below the fourth metacarpal with the flat of the index finger. With the holding hand, grasp the fingers and use the to turn the hand in a clockwise direction several times and a counterclockwise direction several times.

Reposition the flat of the working finger in the area of the wrist below the second metacarpal, the uterus/ prostate reflex area. Grasp the fingers and turn the hand in a clockwise and, then, counterclockwise direction.

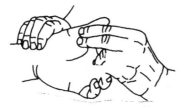

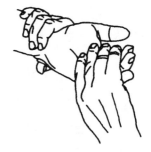

Lateral Surface (Outside) of the Hand

arm

elbow

hand

The arm reflex area runs from the base of the little finger to the fifth metacarpal bone along the outside edge of the hand. In reflex terms, this means that it runs from the neck reflex area to the waistline, as the arm does on the body. The reflex area between the neck and the diaphragm generally corresponds to the upper arm; between the diaphragm and waistline (and even into the knee/ leg reflex area) corresponds to the elbow / forearm / hand.

To apply technique to this reflex area on the left hand, hold the hand vertically. With the left holding hand, stretch the fingers into position. Grasp the fleshy lateral surface of the hand to the outside of the fifth metacarpal bone between the working thumb and index finger. With a simultaneous thumb and finger walking technique application make several passes through the area. Technique may also be applied with the hand held horizontally.

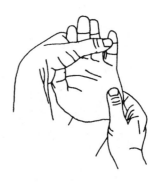

Median Surface (Inside) of the Hand

Spine

Bladder

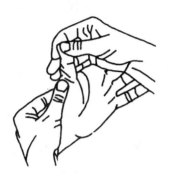

To apply technique to this area, grasp the left thumb with the right holding hand. Holding the thumb steady, walk with the thumb of the left working hand from the radiocarpal joint through the thumb. Change working and holding hands and utilize the thumb walking technique to walk from the thumb tip to the radiocarpal joint.

The base of the thumb serves as the delineator for the cervical vertebrae reflex areas. The base of the first metacarpal serves as the boundary of the tenth thoracic (waistline) reflex area. The carpals represent the lower back and tailbone reflex areas.

Dorsal Surface

The Fingers and Thumb

head / brain / sinus

neck / throat

thyroid / parathyroid

seventh cervical

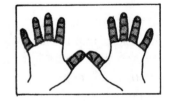

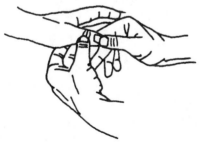

Use the thumb of the holding hand to hold the thumb in place. The fingers of the holding hand act as a brace on the thumb being worked. Walk the thumb in successive passes around the thumb.

Move on to work the fingers. Here the holding hand grasps all four fingers with the thumb and finger tips holding the finger to which technique is applied in place. Walk with the thumb in successive passes around the index finger. Now, reposition the holding hand so that the thumb and finger tips hold the middle finger in place. Use successive passes to cover the finger. Move on to the other two fingers in a similar manner.

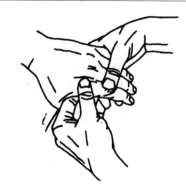

Lung Area and Below on the Dorsal Surface

chest / breast

lung

shoulder

upper back

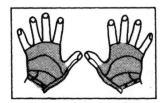

The object here is to work both sides of each of the four troughs on the top of each hand. The hand is held horizontally in front of you. When working the left hand, the right hand most easily serves as the working hand. The holding hand grasps the four fingers to steady the hand. Rest the working thumb at the base of the fingers, in the trough formed by the metacarpal bones. Use the thumb walking technique to work down the length of the metacarpal bone, ending the pass at the carpal bones. Move on to work each trough. Use the right working thumb to walk down the side of the trough formed by the second metacarpal bone.

To work the webbing of the hand and the first metacarpal bone, the left hand most easily serves as the working hand. the right holding hand spreads the thumb and the fingers to form a less fleshy working surface in the web-

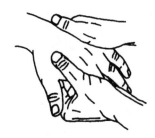

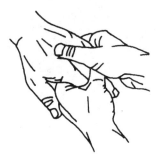

bing of the hand. With the working thumb on the top of the webbing and the working index finger on the palmar surface, use thumb and finger walking simultaneously to make a pass through the area.

The finger walking technique may also be used to work the dorsal surface. The thumb of the working hand rests on the palmar surface to provide leverage for the working finger. Once again, begin work at the base of the finger and walk the length of the metacarpal bone. Work each trough in succession.

Below the Waistline on the Dorsal Surface and Sides

hip / sciatic

hip region

tailbone and spine

lymphatic / groin

hip joint / knee / leg

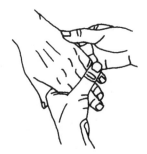

The carpal bones on the dorsal surface of the hand form a bony expanse between the long metacarpal bones and the wrist. To work the area, the left hand serves as a holding hand and the right as the working hand. Begin thumb walking at the base of the fifth metacarpal and thumb walk into the wrist. Make successive passes, beginning thumb walking technique application at the base of each metacarpal. The index finger of the right hand and finger walking technique may also be utilized to work through the area.

Another approach is to grasp the right hand with the right hand as a holding hand. The index finger of the left working hand is utilized to apply finger walking technique across the carpal bones in successive passes. Still another approach is rotating on a point. The index finger of the working hand is placed on top of the hand and the holding hand serves to move the hand being worked in circles. The net result is the exertion of deep pressure. The area represented is below the waistline with its hip, lower back, and pelvic structure. The knee / leg area is located in the carpal area between the fourth and fifth fingers.

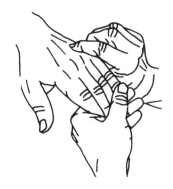

The Wrist (Dorsal Surface): Thumb Walking / Finger Walking / Rotating on a Point

uterus / prostate

ovary / testicle

lymphatic nodes / groin

The uterus/prostate reflex area is located to the medial side of the wrist. It is a pinpoint reflex area located in the gap created by the radiocarpal joint in a straight line below the second metacarpal. To pinpoint the reflex area, place the tip of the working index finger on the wrist. On the left hand, the left index finger most easily serves as a working digit. With the right holding hand, grasp the hand at the base of the fingers. Move the hand in clockwise and then counterclockwise circles using the holding hand.

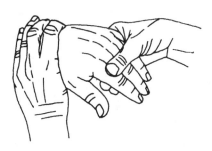

The ovary / testicle reflex area is located to the lateral side of the wrist in a straight line below the fourth metacarpal. To pinpoint the reflex area, place the tip of the working index finger on the wrist. On the left hand, the right index finger most easily serves as a working digit. With the left holding hand, grasp the hand at the base of the fingers. Move the hand in clockwise and then

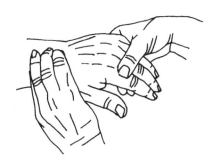

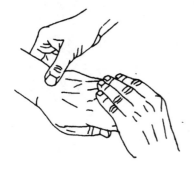

counterclockwise circles using the holding hand.

The thumb walking technique is utilized to apply technique across the entire area. To work the left hand, the left hand serves as a holding hand and the thumb of the right working hand makes several passes across the wrist with the thumb walking technique. Change working and holding hands and work across the wrist from the opposite direction. Finger walking technique may also be utilized in a similar manner.

CHAPTER 7

Movement Techniques

Proprioception literally means to "to perceive oneself". Such perception is possible because of information gathered from muscles, joints, and tendons. The information concerns the stretch of muscles and tendons, the angulation of joints, and deep pressure. From this an image of body position is formed. Standing, for example, is identifiable as a body position different from that of sitting.

Movement technique application is the practice and development of proprioceptive body position not normally experienced in everyday life. In relationship to the hands, movement techniques involve subtle movements. Yet it is those subtle movements that make possible finely tuned activities such as writing or painting. Routine dulls the finely honed edges of the body. Unless the capabilities of the hands are explored, the flexibility and full range of movement are lost. (Use it or lose it.) Movement techniques are a way of developing the hands' potentials. They are an exercise of life's finely tuned movements.

Loss of such abilities can result in the inability to care for oneself. This is a problem with senior citizens which have the ramifications of no longer being able to live independently. For example, the buttoning of buttons, grasp of cooking pots, zipping of zippers, and performance of toilet functions depend upon fingers and hands capable of performing these functions.

Loss of abilities can also result in the inability to participate in life's pleasurable experiences. The painter no longer capable of grasping a brush, the piano player whose finger just won't move, the tennis player whose hands refuse to hold a racket - all are examples of life's little pleasures cut short because of loss of finely tuned hand movement. The application of movement techniques allows for a sharpening of skills in those finely honed capabilities.

The Holding Hand and Working Hand

In movement techniques, the role of the holding hand is a more active one than the holding hand in reflexology pressure technique. The holding hand acts to create appropriate conditions and counter the actions of the working hand. For example, in the pull technique, the working hand grasps and slowly pulls the finger. The holding hand pushes and acts as a counterforce to the pulling of the working hand. The holding hand and working hand act together to accentuate movement. The working hand alone cannot create as much contrast of movement. The hand being worked is supported by resting it on a surface.

In the illustrations, note the placement of the working hand and holding hands that make contact with the client's hand. Such points of contact are illustrated.

Directional Movement of the Hand

To practice movement of the hand in the basic directions of wrist adduction and wrist abduction, grasp the hand at the wrist with the holding hand and at the base of the fingers with the working hand. Push up with the finger tips on the palm of the working hand to move the hand into a position of wrist abduction. Hold for several seconds. Release. Push down with the flat of the thumb of the working hand to move the hand into a position of wrist adduction. Hold for several seconds. Release.

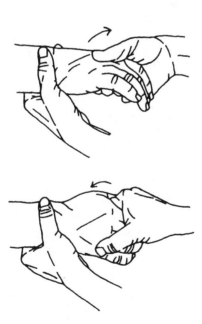

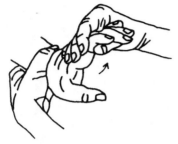 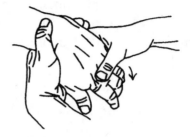

To practice movement of the hand in the basic directions of wrist extension and wrist flexion, grasp the wrist with the holding hand and the fingers with the working hand. Push up with the working thumb, moving the hand up into a position of extension. Hold for several seconds. Release. To practice movement of the hand into a position of flexion, push down with the thumb. Hold for several seconds. Release.

Movement Techniques

Movement techniques create constant, steady movement. Movement is controlled, never sharp or sudden. Controlled movement more closely mimics the subtle actions of a joint. Movement techniques are applied successively to each finger, metacarpal bone or part of the hand.

Note: As in any exercise program, the exercise of the small movements of the hand calls for certain considerations. Start slowly. Proceed cautiously. Do not force any movement. Limit repetitious practice to begin with. Observe individual responses.

Side to Side Movement

The goal of the technique is the practice of a movement of the finger joints that is seldom experienced. The movement is a slight side to side one. The working hand creates the movement, while the holding hand counters the movement by serving as a brace.

The working and holding hands grip the joints of the digit. The flats of the index finger and thumb of the working hand and holding hand serve as levering points. The goal of the technique is the focused movement of the first joint of the thumb by the working hand.

To try the technique, grip the thumb as shown. The right hand in the illustration is the working hand. Move the thumb in the direction of the arrow, pushing with the flat of the working thumb against the flat of the holding index finger. Now move the thumb in a counterdirection, as indicated by the arrow, pushing with the flat of the working index finger against the flat of the holding thumb. Repeat the pattern of movement and counter-movement several times. Go on to the index finger and repeat. Repeat with each finger.

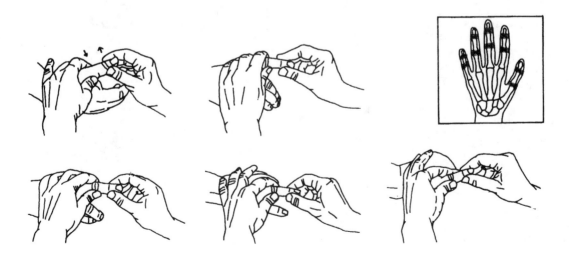

Pull Techniques

The goal of the technique is to allow the fingers and thumb to experience movement in infrequently practiced activity - moving away from the hand. Typically fingers and thumbs spend the day being literally driven towards the body of the hand by activities such as typing.

To practice the pull technique, grasp the thumb with the holding hand (Right hand in illustration.) The holding hand grasps the wrist to isolate the practice of the movement and to counter the actions of the working hand. Pull in a slow, firm movement. Go on to the index finger and repeat. Repeat with each finger.

Variations
Pull and turn technique: With the working hand, pull on the finger and then turn it first in a clockwise direction and them a counterclockwise direction.

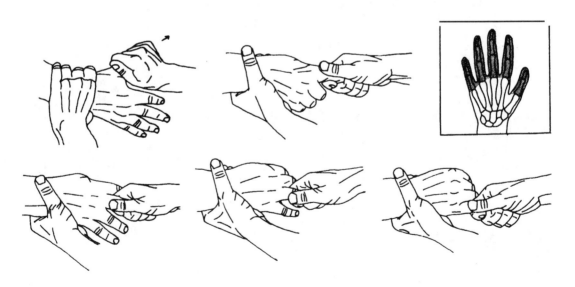

Pull and hold technique: Pull and then turn the finger in a clockwise direction. Hold for a few seconds. Release. Pull, turn in a counterclockwise direction and hold for a few seconds.

Walk Down / Pull Against

The goal of this technique is to create a stretch of the fingers and thumb. While the fingers and thumb have the ability to move slightly in these directions, everyday activities do not make this possible. Aspects of both movement and pressure techniques are utilized. The working thumb is used as a lever against which the fingers pull to create stretch.

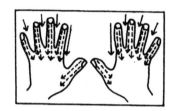

Position the working thumb and fingers as shown. Holding the working thumb in place, pull with the working fingertips against the working thumb tip. The finger is thus placed in a stretched position. Now use the thumb walking technique to walk down the finger. Reposition the working thumb and repeat. As you create a pattern of

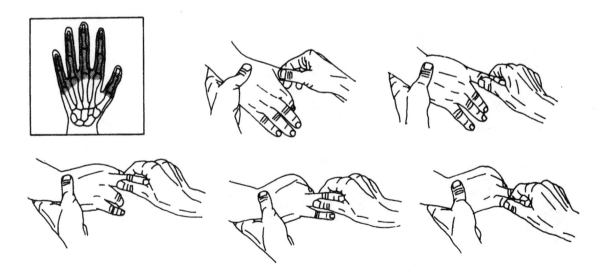

successive passes, note that the finger is stretched from the side in one pass and to the front, away from the palmar surface in another pass.

Metacarpal Lever

The goal of the technique is to work with the metacarpal bones. Once again, a small movement is possible yet seldom experienced in this part of the body.

To try the technique, grasp the hand as shown. The right hand in the illustration is the working hand. Push with the flat of the working thumb. Pull with the flat of the holding index finger to counter the actions of the working thumb. Then, to create movement in a counter direction, pull with the flat of the working index finger and push with the flat of the holding thumb. Repeat the pattern of movement / countermovement several times.

Go on to the next metacarpal bone and repeat. Repeat with each metacarpal bone.

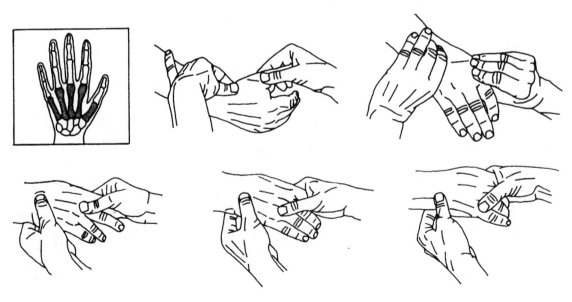

Metacarpal Grasp

The goal of the technique is to create movement between the heads of the metacarpal bones. Grasp the hand as shown. Both hands act as working hands. Push with the flat of the right-hand thumb and pull with the flat of the left-hand index finger. Now, push with the flat of the left-hand thumb and pull with the flat of the right-hand index finger. Repeat the pattern of movement/countermovement several times. Repeat with the other metacarpal bones.

Variation: Move the working and holding hands in circular motions counter to each other.

Variation: Rotate the wrists, pressing the hand with the palms of the working hands. See **1.** Then, counter this movement by rotating the wrist pressing against the hand with the working fingers. See **2.**

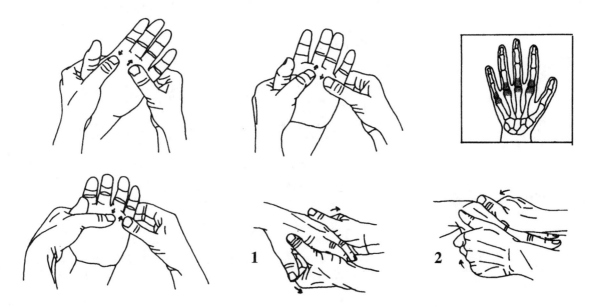

Metacarpal Mover

The object of the technique is to create movement between the metacarpal bones of the hand. First form the working hand into the shape of the grasp.

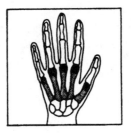 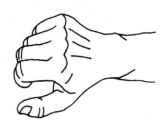

Now, grip the hand with the working hand. The holding hand grips the wrist. The working index finger rests on the top of the hand on the head of the third metacarpal. The working thumb rest on the head of the second metacarpal on the palm of the hand. To create movement, the working index finger pushes against the third metacarpal head, while the working thumb pulls against the second metacarpal head. Leverage is thus create between the two metacarpal heads to promote independent movement.

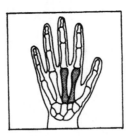 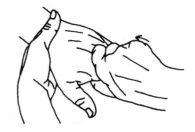

A similar method is used to create movement between the other metacarpals. The working index finger rests of the fourth metacarpal head on top of the hand. The

working thumb rests on the second metacarpal head on
the palm of the hand.

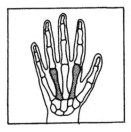 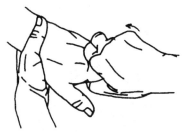

The working index fin-
ger rests on the fifth metacarpal head. The working
thumb remains on the second metacarpal head.

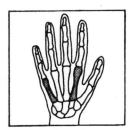 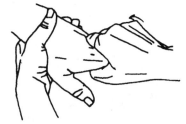

To promote movement
from another direction, a similar technique may be used.
Rest the working thumb on the fourth metacarpal head
on top of the hand. The working index finger rests on the
fifth metacarpal head on the palm of the hand. Push with
the thumb, pull with the finger.
Continue work with

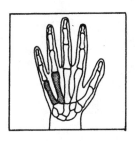 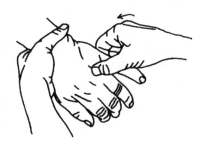

the other metacarpals. Rest the working thumb on the third metacarpal head; the working finger remains on the fifth metacarpal head.

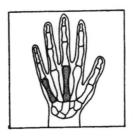 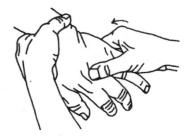

Rest the working thumb on the second metacarpal head; the working index finger remains on the fifth metacarpal head.

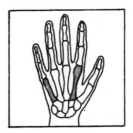 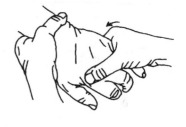

Rest the working thumb on the first metacarpal head; the working index finger remains on the fifth metacarpal head.

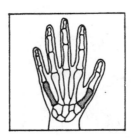 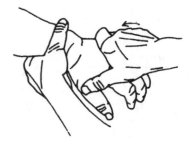

CHAPTER 8

The Technique Session Pattern

The goal of this session pattern is to provide you with an opportunity to present a systematic and thorough application of pressure technique to the entire hand as well as each reflex area. An additional goal is the application of movement techniques both to each and every part of the hand and as desserts between pressure technique application to sections of the hand.

A session includes consideration of client and practitioner comfort in positioning as well as a padded surface for the hand to which technique is applied. Other issues of importance during a session include:
• appropriate use of holding and working hands when applying each technique
• holding and working hands working in concert with each other
• application of successive passes to thoroughly cover a

section of the hand

• smooth transition during change of technique application from one part of the hand to another

• ability to apply technique while not hitting the hand's surface with the fingernail

• maintaining contact with at least one hand on the client's hand at all times

The ability to apply basic techniques adds to the pleasurable experience for the client. Such abilities include:

• use of leverage in the application of thumb walking technique

• appropriate placement of fingers to create leverage for working thumb

• exertion of constant steady pressure in application of finger and thumb walking techniques

• use of the holding hand to create an appropriate surface for the working hand

• application of modified hook and back up technique with minimal fingernail contact

• appropriate placement of working finger to pinpoint reflex area in rotating on a point technique

• slow, steady movement technique application

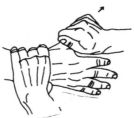

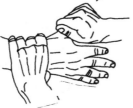

1 Inspect the hand for any cuts, injuries or bruises.

2 Pull technique (Apply to all digits.)

3 Walk down / Pull against (Apply to all digits.)

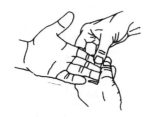

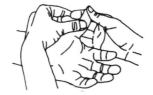

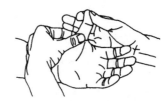

4 Pituitary

5 Head/Brain/Sinus (Apply successive passes.)

6 Neck/Thyroid/Parathyroid (Apply successive passes.)

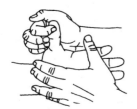

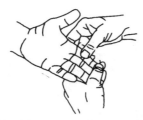

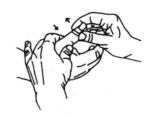

7 Head/Brain/Sinus (Apply successive passes.)

8 Neck/Thyroid/Parathyroid, Teeth/Jaw (Successive passes)

9 Side to side (Apply to all digits.)

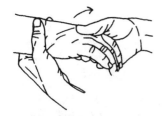

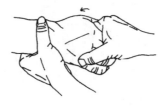

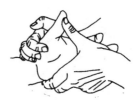

10 Directional movement

11 Directional movement

12 Adrenal gland

105

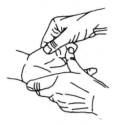

13 Stomach / Pancreas
(Apply successive passes.)

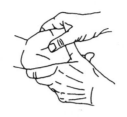

14 Stomach / Pancreas /
Kidney (Successive passes)

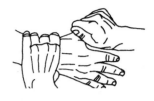

15 Pull technique
(Apply to all digits.)

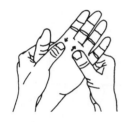

16 Metacarpal grasp
(Apply successive passes.)

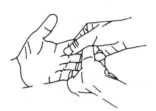

17 Chest / Lung / Breast
(Apply successive passes.)

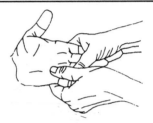

18 Shoulder
(Apply successive passes.)

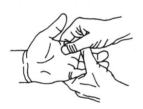

19 Solar plexus / Stomach
(L) / Liver (R)

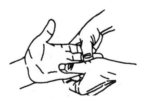

20 Spleen (L) / Liver (R)
(Apply successive passes.)

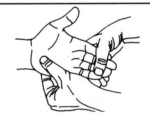

21 Colon / Small intestine
(Apply successive passes.)

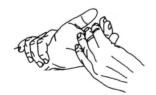

22 Ovary / Testicle

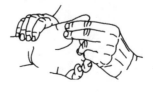

23 Uterus / Prostate

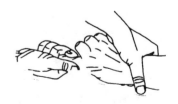

24 Pull technique

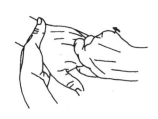

25 Metacarpal mover
(Apply to all.)

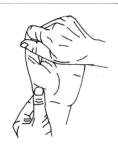

26 Spine
(Apply successive passes.)

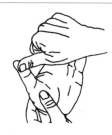

27 Heart
(Apply successive passes.)

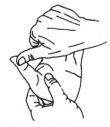

28 Kidney / Stomach
(Apply successive passes.)

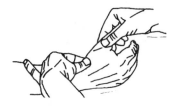

29 Metacarpal lever
(Apply to all.)

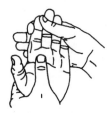

30 Solar plexus / Lung /Chest /
Breast (Apply successive passes.)

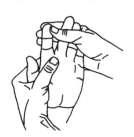

31 Eye /Ear

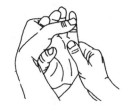

32 Shoulder
(Apply successive passes.)

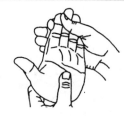

33 Stomach (L) / Liver (R)
(Apply successive passes.)

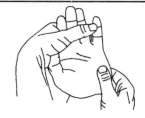

34 Arm / Elbow / Shoulder

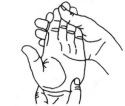

35 Colon / Small intestine

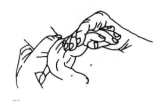

36 Directional movement

107

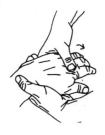

37 Directional movement

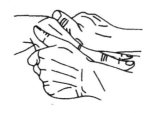

38 Metacarpal grasp

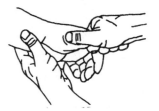

39 Spine

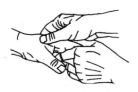

40 Upper back
(Apply successive passes.)

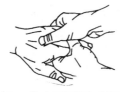

41 Upper back / Chest /
Lung / Breast

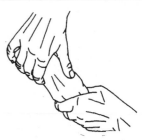

42 Arm / Shoulder

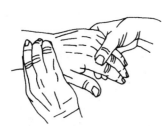

43 Uterus/ Prostate

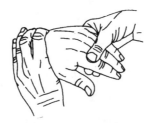

44 Ovary / Testicle

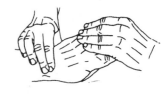

45 Knee / Leg / Lymphatic
nodes / Groin / Fallopian tubes

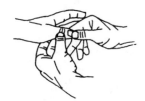

46 Head / Neck

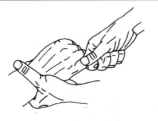

47 Pull

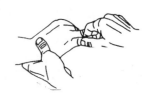

48 Walk down / Pull against

CHAPTER 9

Assessing the Hand

Assessing the hand is a skill acquired by the reflexologist to identify areas of the hand for technique application and/or emphasis. The three-stage process described in this chapter is designed to guide you through an assessment of the stress response of the individual. Assessing the hand is a reading of the stresses the hand and body have experienced. The goal of reading the hand is to (1) Observe and identify stress cues on the hands that indicate the wear-and-tear patterns; (2) Draw inferences from the stress cues to make an evaluation of the adaptation by the hand and body to stress in the terms of reflexology; (3) Elicit from the client feedback about perceptions of what he or she is experiencing as the techniques are applied; and (4) Reach some conclusions about the individual's response to stress.

Observing the Hand

A key element in reading the hand is your ability to observe.

Observing is a process of asking yourself a series of questions that allow you to evaluate the hand. Questions center around stress cues. A stress cue is any part of the hand that shows adaptation to stress. Adaptation to stress is noted through what you observe visibly and with your sense of touch and perception of movement.

Several general rules apply when observing the hand and identifying stress cues. First, observing the hand is a technique of noting and measuring. Noting each stress cue and considering its dimensions provides an opportunity to systematically chronicle the stress pattern of the hand.

Comparing and contrasting is a technique common to identifying any stress cue. The individual's left hand is compared to his or her right hand. This individual's hands are compared to the hands of others. You can, thus, establish a frame of reference to identify stress cues.

Comparing and contrasting is also a part of the questions utilized to identify and evaluate stress cues. For example, when considering the question, "Is this hand puffy?" the answer is "Yes, compared to other hands, it is puffy." Or, "No, compared to other hands, it isn't puffy."
Look for the noteworthy when observing the hands. For example, consider the question, "Which is the most significant, noteworthy characteristic of this particular hand?" Or, consider a question such as, "Is this the thinnest hand I've ever seen?" Or, "Is this the most callousing I've seen on any hand?" If your answer to yourself is 'yes' to any such question, it is a hand with a stress cue to which you will compare future hands and stress cues you will observe. Also, it is a stress cue that can act as a frame of reference for assessment of the individual's hand.

Take into consideration normal use when observing any hand. The hand of a sixty-year-old is not the hand of a twenty-year-old. A certain number of stress cues can be expected with the wear and tear of stress over the years. The hand is observed within its context. Observations are made such as, "This hand shows signs of stress adaptation but, all things considered, not as many as I would expect."

Observe the individual's hands at rest. Are the fingers curled? How curled? Are they stretched out and relaxed? Restless and drumming? Are the fingers of both hands curled equally? Relaxed? Restless? Does the individual wear rings, a watch or bracelets? Several rings? Heavy rings, watch or bracelets?

To practice observing the hand and identifying stress cues, observe a variety of hands. Compare young hands to older hands. Compare men's hands to women's hands. With practice, you will learn to quickly identify stress cues that signify targets and indicate target strategies for your technique application.

We have organized a systematic observation of the hand into four basic techniques: observing visual stress cues, observing touch stress cues, observing sensitivity stress cues, and observing movement stress cues. We have selected particular vocabulary words such as puffiness, thickness, and hard tonus to serve as terms to describe stress cues and note gradations of stress. Somewhat puffy?

Do the hands appear to have areas of **thickness** or texture that is well-padded and dense? Where? How thick is the area? How large is the thick area? Is the whole hand thick? Somewhat thick?

Do you see **callousing** on the hand anywhere? Where? In several areas? How thick is the callousing? How large is the calloused area? Is the entire bottom of the hand calloused? Are the callouses hard? Clear? Shiny? Yellow? Cracked?

Observing Visual Stress Cues

Observing visual signs of stress on the hand involves noting the visible surface of the hand. Just as the surface of the hand has its visible stress landmarks, the surface of the hand too is notable for its signs of adaptation to stress. To observe the hand in more detail, begin with the fingernails and proceed on to the fingers, ball of the hand, body, the heel, and the top of the hand in a systematic manner.

Consider the following commonly found stress cues. Visually observable hand stress is described in terms of texture, hand features, and color. Can you find any of these characteristics of stress on the hand you are observing?

Texture

Texture observations are made to note the surface character of the hand. The goal is to observe any adaptation to stress that appears on the surface of the hand. Texture is described in terms of *thinness, puffiness, thickness, muscularity,* and *callousing.*

Observe the hand in general. What is your impression of the hand? Is it a thin hand? A thick hand? A muscular hand? Is the surface of the hand consistent in texture? What do you consider the most outstanding visual characteristic of the hand? Do you note several outstanding characteristics? Do the characteristics center around one part of the hand?

Do you see **puffiness** on the hand anywhere? Where? How puffy is it? How large is the puffy area? Are there several puffy areas? Is the surface of the hand puffy?

Visual Stress Cures

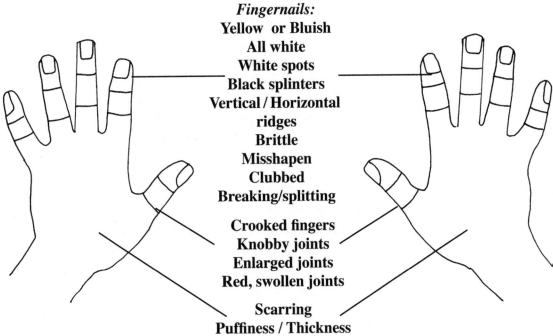

Texture:
Thin hand
Thick hand
Muscular hand
Consistent

Stress lines

Puffiness
Thickness
Callousing
Scarring

Color:
Natural
White speckling
Very red
Very white

Fingernails:
Yellow or Bluish
All white
White spots
Black splinters
Vertical / Horizontal
ridges
Brittle
Misshapen
Clubbed
Breaking/splitting

Crooked fingers
Knobby joints
Enlarged joints
Red, swollen joints

Scarring
Puffiness / Thickness

Hand Feature

A hand feature is a distinctive or outstanding visual landmark on the hand. A hand feature indicates a structure of the hand itself that has been altered by adaptation to stress. Several of these stress cues are also considered hand problems.

Observe the hand in general. Do you note any distinctive or outstanding hand features? Are there several hand features? Do both the right and the left hand show the same hand features?

Do you note **scarring** anywhere on the hands?

Are the fingers **straight** in appearance? Are any **crooked?** How many? How crooked? At which finger joint does the bend occur? Are the fingers of both hands crooked?

Are the joints of the fingers **normal and uniform** in size? Are any of them *enlarged*? Red and swollen? Which one(s)? Do any show signs of injury, such as scarring, diminution in size or stiffness?

Are the fingernails **regularly shaped**? Irregularly you feel, the nature of the hand itself, is directly linked to the stress the hand has experienced. As a rule of thumb, the puffier, the thicker, the harder the tonus, the more adaptation to stress has taken place over time. Also, the pattern of stress is more deeply ingrained as a learning experience, and a longer time period will be required to condition the hand with pressure technique.

Touch cues are described in terms of tonus, or the resistance to pressure technique application, as perceived by the reflexologist. **Puffiness, thickness, hard tonus, callousing,** and **stringiness** are terms utilized to note qualities and gradations of the felt surface. Hand temperature evaluation is a further touch assessment technique.

shaped? Are they brittle and split? Do any show signs of injury such as irregular shape or a partial nail?

What **color** are the nails? Pink/white? Yellow? Bluish? Pure white? Are all uniform in color? Do any or all show vertical ridges? Horizontal ridges? Spots of white? Small black splinter-like areas underneath?

Are the joints at the base of the fingers enlarged?

Do you see **stress lines** (lines other than those relating to the palm print) on the palmar surface of the hands? In the fingers? In the thenar eminence?

Color

Observing the **color** of the hand is a matter of noting the consistency of skin tone. While color does not necessarily show circulatory stress, color serves as a general indicator of circulation. A very white hand shows a lack of circulation to the hand. A very red hand indicates a lack of circulation from the hand. A blue hand shows a lack of oxygen. White speckling shows an interruption in circulation.

Observe the hand. Is the **skin tone** of the hand natural in color? Is the color of the hand uniform? Is there any white speckling? Where? Over how large an area? Is the whole hand very white? Very red? Cyanotic (blue)?

Observing the Touch Stress Cue

Observing the touch stress cue involves noting the feel of the hand as thumb and finger walking techniques are applied. More than any other stress cue, the cue of touch provides a valuable asset to the reflexologist. When you apply technique to the hand, what do you feel? What

Touch Stress Cues

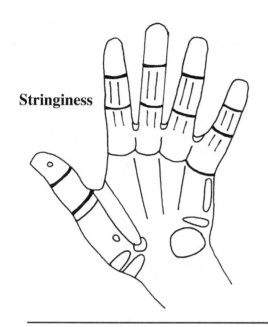

Stringiness

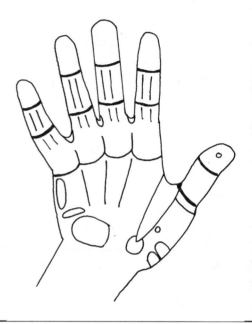

Temperature:
Hot
Cold
Perspiring

Puffiness
Thickness
Lack of tonus
Hard tonus
Callousing

Sensitivity

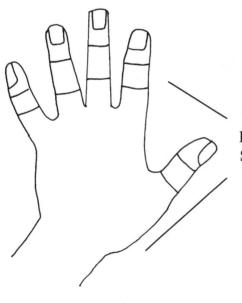

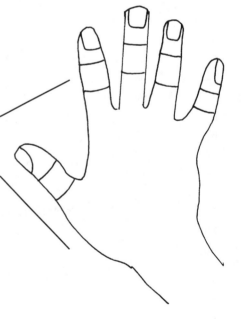

Puffiness
Thickness
Hard tonus
Stringiness

116

As you work through the hand, compare your touch observations in one part of the hand to the others. For example, does the ball of the hand show the same touch characteristics as the heel of the hand? Then, is the whole hand uniform in its feel? Do both hands show the same touch characteristics?

Begin your touch observations with the application of the thumb walking technique to the ball of the hand. Go on to apply this technique to fingers, ball of the hand, thenar eminence, the body, the heel, and the top of the hand. Some of the touch stress cues share the same name as visual stress cues. Be sure to make a touch observation of the visual cues of the same name you have observed. The touch observation is added to your visual observation. As you apply technique to the hand, do you observe any of the following stress cues?

Is there a feeling of **puffiness** when you apply thumb walking technique to any part of the hand? Does the surface under your thumb feel soft and spongy? Fluidlike? Puffy with some resistance to pressure? Puffy with a stringy band? Where is the puffiness? Over how large an area? The whole hand? How does the puffiness contrast with the surrounding area? Is the surrounding area somewhat puffy? Different in tone?

Do you feel solid resistance, a **thickness**, when you apply pressure to any part of the hand? Where? How thick is it? Does it have a distinctive shape? Over how large an area? The whole hand? Does the hand feel somewhat thick all over? When you apply technique to the hand, do you feel a uniformity of thickness?

Do you note an area **lacking tonus**? Where? How thin is it? Over how large an area? Is it distinctive over a portion of the hand? Is there a sharp contrast between the area lacking tonus and the surrounding area? Is the entire hand lacking tonus?

Do you feel an area of concentrated hardness? Where? Over how large an area? What is the shape of the area? Is the **hard tonus** surrounded by thick tonus? Puffiness? Callousing? Is there a sharp contrast between the area of hard tonus and the surrounding area? Do you find a variety of touch stress cues ranging from puffiness to thickening to thickened to hardened?

When you apply pressure technique to a calloused part of the hand, what do you feel? Do you feel thickness? Hardness? Is the **callousing** somewhat hard? Hard with a surrounding area of thickness? How large an area is calloused? Is there a distinctive shape to the callousing? If there are several calloused areas on the hand, are they uniform in callousing?

When applying pressure technique to any part of the hand, do you feel **stringiness** or a resistance to pressure over a stringlike area? Does the stringiness feel like a thin wire or a thick rope?

What is your initial impression of the hand's **temperature**? Is the hand hot or cold to the touch initially? **Perspiring?** (A warmer than usual hand shows an overly active circulatory system. A cooler than usual hand indicates an under-active circulatory system or interruption in circulation from the neck. A perspiring hand shows an over-active elimination system.)

Do both hands show the same or similar touch stress cues? Do both hands show a concentration of touch stress cues in the same parts of the hand, such as the fingers?

Observing Sensitivity and Client Comments as Stress Cues

As the reflexologist works with a client's hands, the client frequently responds to technique application with a comment. Comments range from reports of sensitivity to observations about perceived feelings resulting from technique applied to a particular area of the hand.

The reflexologist asks "How does that feel to you?" when encountering an extreme visual or touch stress cue or a response from the client such as, "What's that?" By eliciting and clarifying client feedback, the reflexologist better assesses the client's stress pattern.

A client is less likely to respond to pressure applied to the hands with a report of sensitivity than during pressure applied to the feet. Hands are unprotected during their day to day activities while feet are protected by shoes and thus more sensitive. Typical sensitivity responses include: It's dull pain. It's sharp pain. It's dull with tingling. It's sharp with tingling. It hurts but it hurts good. It hurts bad. It's too much.

Reports of sensitivity generally occur in two locations on the hand: (1) pinpoint areas of the hand when deep pressure is applied and (2) aging joints of the fingers when a pressure or movement technique is applied, especially to red or swollen joints.

It is not unusual to receive a response of sensitivity to the application of pressure to pinpoint areas. While hands in general are exposed to pressure throughout the day, areas that are pinpointed are buried in padded areas of the hands. They do not frequently receive pressure sensation and an area of pinpoint sensitivity is indicative of a stress.
Reports of sensitivity in response to movement of joints, however, may indicate an old injury, a recent injury or an arthritic condition. Avoidance is the best policy. Future work may be considered when the joint is less sensitive.
In either of the above situations, your evaluation of the sensitivity continues with a comparison of the sensitivity to the other stress cues in the area. What did the sensitive area feel like to

you? Are there visual and touch stress cues? How large an area is sensitive? From what you feel, are you surprised at the level of sensitivity or is it about what you would expect considering the hand stress?

Observing Movement Technique Cues

Observation of cues during the application of movement techniques includes noting the ease of movement, the range of the movement, and any report of sensitivity.

Techniques Applied to the Fingers

During the application of the side to side technique, the practitioner's hands create a small movement at the joints of the finger. Is noise produced when any of the joints is moved? Which one(s)? Does the joint show signs of visual stress cues? Does the individual comment on the sound or about sensitivity during movement? Observe the degree of movement possible when technique is applied to each of the individual's digits. Are the digits and joints uniform in degree of movement? If not, which are unique? Do these digits or joints show signs of visual stress cues?

During the application of the walk down/pull against technique, the practitioner's hands create a stretch of the finger as a whole or a stretch at the joints of the finger. Observe the degree of stretch possible when technique is applied to each of the individual's digits. Are the digits and joints uniform in degree of stretch? If not, which are unique? Do these digits or joints show signs of visual stress cues? Does the individual comment about sensitivity during the stretch? Does the joint show signs of visual stress cues?

During the application of the pull technique, the practitioner creates a stretch of the finger and body of the hand. Does the individual report pain, discomfort or feelings of stress in response?

During the application of movement techniques to the body of the hand (metacarpal lever, metacarpal grasp, and metacarpal mover), the practitioner's hands create a stretch and movement of the hand in directions not commonly found during everyday activities. Movement is encouraged by action taken on the metacarpal heads of the individual's hands. Observe the degree of movement possible when technique is applied to the metacarpal heads. Is the movement uniform between each pair of metacarpal heads when technique is applied? If not, which are unique? Does the body of the hand or the metacarpal head show signs of visual stress cues? Does the individual comment about sensitivity during the stretch or movement?

CHAPTER 10

Drawing Inferences from Stress Cues

Evaluating the Hand

How stressed is a particular hand? This is the basic question that you should keep in mind while evaluating the hand. An image of the hand's stress pattern helps you determine a plan of action. The stress cue is the basic building block in constructing an image of stress patterns. The absence of a stress cue, the presence of a stress cue, and the characteristics of the stress cues are used to create fairly predictable inferences about stress.

The characteristics of the stress cue provide you with a means of measuring stress. The magnitude of the stress cue, its location, and the level of the client's stress awareness all provide information you can develop into a technique strategy that most effectively and efficiently relaxes the stress of a particular individual.

The Basic Rule of Hand Stress / Relaxation is
The more the adaptation to stress over a longer period of

time: (1) The more extreme the stress cue, (2) The more deeply ingrained the pattern of stress and the disturbance within reflexes, (3) The greater the potential for the individual's awareness of stress and stress-related problems, (4) The more conditioning by pressure technique application will be required over a longer period of time to change the pattern of stress.

In making an assessment, you reach conclusions about the impact of stress on the hand and the body. Three basic techniques measure stress response: (1) The Hand Stress Scale describes the range along which stress adaptation takes place on the hand, (2) The Reflex Stress Scale describes the range of stress adaptation reflected in the hand's reflexes, (3) The Body Stress Scale provides an opportunity for the reflexologist to compare his or her findings about stress adaptation to the individual's feelings about his or her stress level.

Evaluating the Hand Stress Pattern

The presence of a hand stress cue indicates an adaptation to stress. In evaluating hand stress cues, the reflexologist measures stress by considering the characteristics of the stress cue. The measurement is in terms of adaptation to stress. The terms *alarm*, *adaptation*, and *exhaustion* parallel those of Selye and his stress theory. Such generalized terms create a scale by which to evaluate the impact of stress.

In the *alarm stage of adaptation*, the stress cue shows signs of a lesser stress that has been adapted to over a shorter period of time or a stress that has little impact. If the stress is a recent event, the body is in the process of learning how to cope, and a lesser amount of technique application will be required to cause a change in stress level. Immediate change is possible because the stress pattern is not deeply ingrained, and merely interrupt-

123

ing the stress can reshape and condition the stress pattern. Another possibility: In the *alarm stage of adaptation,* the hand may be sensitive to very sensitive to untouchable in response to pressure technique application. The hand thus shows signs of an immediate stress being adapted to by the body right now. It can be (1) a short-term stress of such magnitude as to register ponderable disturbance or (2) a long-term, chronic stress that is currently active and acute.

In the *adaptive stage*, the stress cue shows signs of a stress adapted to over a period of time that has created some impact. The stress has been ingrained as a learning experience. Another possibility: A recent stress of some magnitude has caused the body to adapt to considerable stress quickly. In either case, consistency of technique application over time will be required to cause a change in stress level. Some immediate change may be possible as technique application interrupts stress sufficiently to cause a shift in the stage of adaptation.

In the *exhaustion stage of adaptation*, the stress cue shows signs of a stress adapted to over a lengthy time period. The stress has been deeply ingrained as a learning experience. Another possibility: A recent stress of considerable magnitude has occurred, such as a serious accident, injury, illness, or emotional stress. Either will require regular technique application over a length of time to produce long-term results. Immediate change is possible as technique application interrupts current stress. A shift in stage of adaptation is possible over time.

Evaluating the Hand Stress Cue

In making hand stress inferences, the reflexologist considers the characteristics of the stress cue. Not only is a stress cue described as, for example, a crooked finger, but the quality of crookedness is also measured and graded. The net result is accurate rating of the stage of adaptation. In addition, further inferences about stress patterns can be drawn.

To practice making inferences, once again (1) Consider the hand you have observed in the previous section, (2) Consider each stress cue that you observed, and (3) See if you can match it to a description of a stage of adaptation on the Hand Stress Scale. The left-hand column lists the stress cues. The other columns list the three stages of adaptation with stress cue characteristics listed under each. Select the stress cue and then find the column that best describes the characteristics you have found in that stress cue.

Making Hand Stress Inferences

Once you have assessed each stress cue individually, consider the overall pattern of adaptation. Are most of the stress cues listed in the same column; thus, in the same stage of adaptation? Or are they of varied stages of adaptation? Are many of the stress cues gathered in one part of the hand, such as in the fingers? Do the various parts of the hand differ in stages of adaptation?

These further inferences provide more depth to your evaluation. A stress cue that shows an adaptive level of other stress cues may be an indicator of an isolated stress incident, such as an accident or a hand injury. Stress cues that share adaptive level throughout only one part of the hand, such as the fingers, are an indicator of a particular pattern of stress. Stress cues of similar levels throughout the hand show the overall level of stress adaptation.

Once again, consider the hand. What is your assessment of the overall pattern of adaptation by the hand? Is it the same as the level of adaptation by the other hand?

Consider each stress cue observed in the previous section. Match each to the level of adaptation as noted in the following chart.

Hand Stress Scale

Stress Cue	Level of Stress Adaptation		
	Alarm	**Adaptation**	**Exhaustion**
Visual Stress Cues			
Texture	Puffiness	Thickness	callousing
Hand Feature	Scarring	Older scar	Older scar, wide area
	Finger somewhat crooked	Very crooked	Misshapen
	Finger joint irregular	Enlarged	Red, swollen
	Fingernail shape irregular, brittle, injured	Several in number or very irregular, brittle, injured	All extremely irregular, brittle, injured
	Fingernail color not uniform or yellow, bluish, pure white	Very unusual coloring	Extreme unusual coloring
	Fingernail horizontal ridges, vertical ridges, spots of white, black splinter-like areas	Several fingernails with ridges, spots, black splinter-like areas	Extreme ridges, spots of white, black splinter-like areas
	Stress lines	Over area, deep	Over wide area/very deep
Color	Some white speckling	Wide area white speckling	Whole hand very white, red, or blue
Touch Stress Cues	Puffiness	Thickness	Hard tonus, callousing
	Cool, warm	Cold sometime, hot sometime	Very cold all the time, very hot all the time, perspiring
Sensitivity Stress Cues	Sharp, little tone	Sharp, deep	Aching, wide area
Movement Stress Cues	Some resistance	Stiff	Immovable

Evaluating the Reflex Stress Pattern

How stressed is a particular reflexive area or region? This is the basic question asked by the reflexologist in assessing the hand's reflex areas. The location and patterns of the stress cue are the basic building blocks to construct an image of reflexive stress patterns. Again, the characteristic of the stress cue provides certain predictable features. The location of a stress cue is assessed according to the reflex area chart. The chart is a map of the body's plan for adaptation to stress as it relates to body parts. The reflex chart tells you where to look for stress cues and patterns of stress cues.

Evaluating the Reflex Stress Cue

How do you know when adaptation to stress by the reflexes has taken place? Counting stress cues, noting location, and assessing the adaptive level of each provides a picture of the reflex stress pattern

The terms used to describe the pattern of reflex stress are *local, regional,* and *general.* A *local* pattern of reflex stress is indicated by a small concentrated area of stress cues, such as two or more stress cues in any one reflex area OR one or more exhausted or extremely sensitive stress cues in any one reflex area

A *regional* pattern of reflex stress is indicated by a concentration of stress cues throughout a part of the hand such as the fingers, three or more alarm stress cues, two or more adapted stress cues, one or more exhausted stress cues in the fingers

Stress cues throughout every part of the hand indicate a *generalized* pattern of reflex stress. A generalized pattern is reflected by two or more regions in any one hand showing adaptation, such as the fingers and the heel of the hand; one or more regions showing exhaustion; two or more extremely sensitive regions; a majority of the glands or organs within a system showing stress cues, such as three of the five endocrine glands or three or more stressed reflex areas within a zone.

Making Reflex Stress Inferences

The Reflex Stress Scale has been developed to provide a basic technique of reflex stress assessment. The left-hand column lists the possible location of stress cues. The right-hand columns list the number of stress cues and the stage of adaptation of the stress cues.

A reflex stress inference is made by considering the pattern of stress cues. The location, type (stage of adaptation), and number of stress cues combine together to indicate the pattern of stress. A reflexive stress pattern is established if a sufficient number of stress cues of a particular magnitude are present.

To practice this technique, consider the stress cues on a hand. (1) Count the exhausted stress cues, the adapted stress cues, and the alarm stress cues. (2) Consider the location of each stress cue. (3) Tally up the type, number, and location of stress cues. (4) Create a reference chart similar to the one shown as the Reflex Stress Scale.

Reflex Stress Scale

Consider the stress cues on the hand. Consider the type of stress cue, such as alarm, and the location of each. Tally up the type, number, and location of the stress cues to create a picture of the pattern of stress, such as local, regional, or general.

Location of Stress Cue	Reflex Areas: Number and Type of Stress Cues		
	Number of Alarm Stress Cues	Number of Adapted Stress Cues	Number of Exhausted Stress Cues

Local Pattern of Stress
A local pattern of adaptation to stress has occurred if there is a total of:

	2 or more in any one reflex area	2 or more in any one reflex area	1 or more in any one reflex area OR 1 extremely sensitive reflex area

Regional Pattern of Stress
A regional pattern of adaptation to stress has occurred if there is a total of:

Fingers	3 or more	2 or more	1 or more
Ball of hand	3 or more	2 or more	1 or more
Body of hand	3 or more	2 or more	1 or more
Heel of hand	3 or more	2 or more	1 or more
Top of hand	3 or more	2 or more	1 or more

General Pattern of Stress
A general adaptation to stress has occurred if there is a total of:

Regions (See above)		2 or more	1 or more OR 2 or more extremely sensitive regions

Location of Stress Cue	Reflex Areas: Number and Type of Stress Cues		
	Number of Alarm Stress Cues	**Number of Adapted Stress Cues**	**Number of Exhausted Stress Cues**

General Pattern of Stress
A systematic adaptation to stress has occurred if there is a total of:

Location of Stress Cue	Number of Alarm Stress Cues	Number of Adapted Stress Cues	Number of Exhausted Stress Cues
Endocrine System (Pituitary, adrenal glands, pancreas, thyroid/parathyroid, ovary/testicle, uterus/prostate)	3 of the 5 endocrine reflex areas	2 of the 5 endocrine reflex areas	1 or more of the 5 endocrine reflex areas
Digestive System (Stomach, gallbladder, liver, pancreas, small intestine, large intestine)	3 of the 6 digestive reflex areas	2 of the 6 digestive reflex areas	1 or more of the 6 digestive reflex areas
Musculo-skeletal System (Shoulder, neck, back, arm, elbow, hip, leg, knee, ankle, wrist, hand, foot)	3 musculo-skeletal reflex areas	2 musculo-skeletal reflex areas	1 musculo-skeletal reflex area
Urinary System (Kidneys, bladder)	2 of the 2 urinary reflex areas	1 of the 2 urinary reflex areas	1 of the 2 urinary reflex areas
Reproductive System (Ovary/uterus/fallopian tubes (for women), Testicle/prostate (for men))	3 of 3 of the reproductive reflex areas (women) 2 of 2 (men)	2 of 3 of the reproductive reflex areas (women) 1 of 2 (men)	1 of 3 of the reproductive reflex areas (women) 1 of 2 (men)
Lymphatic System (Lymphatic gland, visual stress cues)	lymphatic gland reflex area, puffiness	lymphatic gland reflex areas, puffiness	lymphatic gland reflex areas, puffiness
Respiratory System (Lungs)	lung reflex area	lung reflex area	lung reflex area
Cardio-vascular system (Heart)	heart reflex area	heart reflex area	heart reflex area

130

Location of Stress Cue	Reflex Areas: Number and Type of Stress Cues		
	Number of Alarm Stress Cues	Number of Adapted Stress Cues	Number of Exhausted Stress Cues
Circulatory System (Visual stress cues)	color, puffiness	color, puffiness	color, puffiness
Nervous System (solar plexus, brain, spine)	3 of 3 reflex areas	2 of 3	1 or more

General Pattern of Stress
A zonal adaptation to stress has occurred if there is a total of:

Zone 1 (Head/neck/sinus, thyroid/parathyroid/ throat, eyes, teeth, lymphatic duct, thymus, chest/lung, heart, solar plexus, liver, adrenal glands, pancreas, stomach, colon, small intestine, bladder, spine from neck to tailbone)	3 reflex areas in the zone	2 reflex areas in the zone	1 reflex area in the zone
Zone 2 (Head/neck/sinus, teeth, eyes, chest/lung, heart, solar plexus, liver (right), pancreas (left), stomach (left), kidneys, small intestine, lower back)	3 reflex areas	2 reflex areas	1 reflex area
Zone 3 (Head/neck/sinus, teeth, inner ear, chest/ lung, liver (right), kidneys, small intestine, lower back)	3 reflex areas	2 reflex areas	1 reflex area
Zone 4 (Head/neck/sinus, teeth, ears, shoulder/ chest, liver /gallbladder (right), colon, small intestine, lower back)	3 reflex areas	2 reflex areas	1 reflex area

Location of Stress Cue	Reflex Areas: Number and Type of Stress Cues		
	Number of Alarm Stress Cues	**Number of Adapted Stress Cues**	**Number of Exhausted Stress Cues**
Zone 5 (Head/neck/sinus, jaw, ears, shoulder joint, liver, colon, ileocecal valve, hip/ knee, lower back)	3 reflex areas	2 reflex areas	1 reflex area

Evaluating the Body Stress Pattern

How stressed is this individual and how aware is he or she of his or her stress level? The reflexologist focuses on such questions about body stress by (1) listening to the individual or (2) asking questions of the individual. Both methods help the reflexologist confirm, refute, or change his or her assessment of the impact of stress on the individual. These responses and general comments are measured against your own findings.

The technique of interviewing an individual about his or her stress response takes practice. The skill is in asking the questions.

1. Asking too many questions will interrupt the relaxation provided by the session and give the individual the false perception that you have found problems that he or she should worry about. Ask a minimal amount of questions. Your goal is to gauge the impact of stress on the individual and to determine a stage of adaptation.

2. Ask questions of a broad, general nature. A question that is phrased, "Does your neck bother you?" is of a broad, general nature. It allows the individual to respond in a variety of ways: How long the stress has been present; what impact they're feel-

ing, if any; and whether they consider it a problem. A follow-up question such as, "How long has it bothered you?" or "Do you consider it a problem?" will fill in the gaps of information you need to evaluate the hand.

Evaluating Body Stress Cues

A question is prompted by stress cues of such magnitude or number they show that adaptation to stress has taken place. The purpose of the questions is to identify the pattern of adaptation within the individual's stress mechanism. There are two basic responses to a question such as "Does your neck bother you?" – yes and no.

Yes tells you that the individual is feeling the impact of stress and further questions or their comments will fill in the picture.

"Yes, right now." The individual is reporting that he or she is bothered by a stressed reflex area, reflex region, or stress-related condition currently.

"Yes, once in a while." The individual is reporting that he or she feels the effects of a stress occasionally. This indicates a stress pattern of less wear and tear that has not been deeply ingrained. Keep in mind, however, that the individual may not be accurately reporting his or her stress adaptation. It may be deeply ingrained but overridden by the individual.

"Yes, it comes and goes." The individual is reporting that the stress recurs on a regular basis. It is ingrained to the point that the wear- and-tear pattern is becoming conditioned as a stress response. The individual's ability to rebound from a stress event such as an illness takes place within limits.

"Yes, all the time." The individual is reporting that he or she feels the effects of chronic stress.The wear-and-tear pattern of stress has ingrained itself over a lengthy time period. If the individual names a disorder or reports a diagnosis, the stress

response has been present long enough to acquire a name such as "my neck problem" or "The doctors tell me I have scoliosis." Also, a report of a stress event such as a car accident, operation, illness, or emotional distress is a clue to possible extensive wear and tear.

No can have several meanings and can tell you something about the individual's perception of stress and his or her ability to cope with it.

"No, it doesn't bother me." By giving a negative response to a single question about a stress cue on the hand, the individual, thus, is reporting that impact of the stress is negligible and he or she has the ability to cope with the stress.

"No, it did bother me." By giving this response, the individual is reporting that he or she is not aware of the stress at this time and has learned to adapt and cope with the stress.

"No, nothing really bothers me." By giving a negative response to almost every question, this individual may be unaware of the effects of stress altogether. The individual has learned to cope by overriding his or her stress mechanism. Continuous overstressing can lead to exhaustion.

Body Stress Scale

Consider asking a question if any stress cue is of sufficient magnitude to draw your attention or if any pattern of stress cues draws your attention. This chart should serve only as a guide and not as a diagnostic tool.

Fingers

A. Do you ever have headaches or problems with your upper back or neck?

1. Do you have headaches?

2. Do your sinuses bother you? Do you have sinus headaches?

3. Does your neck bother you?

4. Does your jaw bother you?

5. Do you have teeth problems?

Webbing of fingers

B. Do your eyes and ears bother you?

6. Do your ears bother you?

7. When you get up quickly, do you occasionally get dizzy?

8. Do your eyes bother you?

9. Do you feel tension on the tops of your shoulders?

Thenar eminence / ball of the hand

C. Have you ever had problems in the back or chest region?

10. Do you feel tension in the upper back? Chest?

11. Do you feel tension between the shoulder blades?
   In the chest? In the neck? Upper back?

12. Do you feel tension between the shoulder blades?

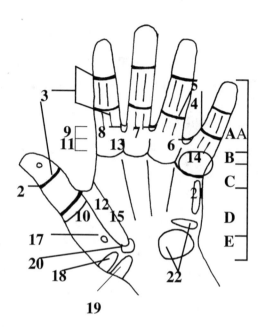

13. Do you get heavy chest colds in the winter?

14. Does your shoulder bother you?

15. Are you under a lot of stress?

16. Do you get acid indigestion?

17. Do you have allergies? Asthma? Hay fever? Sinus problems? Feelings of total exhaustion?

18. Do you experience sudden drops in energy? In the afternoon?

19. Does your stomach bother you?

20. Have you had problems with your kidneys?

Body of the hand

D. Does your midback to lower back ever bother you?

21. Does your arm bother you?

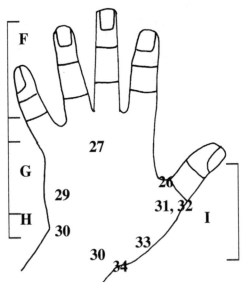

Heel

E. Does your lower back bother you?

22. Do you have digestive problems?

23. Does your lower back bother you?

24. Have you injured your lower back?

25. Do you have digestive problems? Lower back problems?

Top of hand

Fingers

F. Does your neck bother you?

G. Does your chest or upper back bother you?

26. Do you get numbness in the fingers? Do your hands get cold?

27. Do you feel tension in the upper back or chest?

28. Do you have digestive problems?

29. Does your knee, hip, leg or lower back bother you?

Wrist

H. Do your legs and hips ever bother you?

30. Have you had reproductive problems?

Inside of hand

I. Does your back bother you?

31. Does your neck bother you?

32. Do you feel tension between the shoulder blades?

33. Does your back bother you, particularly in the middle?

34. Does your lower back bother you?

CHAPTER 11

The Assessment Session

Once again, reading the hand is a skill acquired by the reflexologist to identify areas of the hand for technique application emphasis. The information you gather through reading the hand serves as a gauge for technique application, a reference point to measure change, and an indicator of stress priorities.

Reading the hand allows the reflexologist to reach some conclusions about the individual's response to stress. Two qualities of stress response are noted: (1) the level of adaptation, such as alarm, adaptation, or exhaustion, and (2) the type of response, such as hand stress, reflex stress, or body stress. Thus, the hand, the reflex, and the body can be evaluated for stress.

Reading the Hand: Session Pattern

The following session pattern provides you with an

opportunity to practice observing and evaluating the hand in a systematic manner. Each segment is organized with visual stress cue observations first, then touch / sensitivity, followed by press and assess stress cue observations. A summary of observations and an evaluation of hand, reflex, and body stress inferences completes the segment. The goal of the completed session pattern is to create an assessment of the individual's pattern of stress. This session pattern should serve only as a guide and not a diagnostic tool.

(1) Observe the hand as you look it over for cuts, callouses, and bruises. What is your general impression of the hand? Is it a thick hand? A thin hand? An average hand? What do you consider the most outstanding visual cue on the hand? Are there several significant cues? Do the visual cues center around one part of the hand, such as the ball of the hand? How does this hand compare in general to the hands of individuals of the same gender and age group? Does the hand show what you might expect with respect to stress cues?

The Fingers

head / brain / sinus

pituitary / hypothalamus

jaw / teeth / gums

thyroid / parathyroid

neck / throat / seventh cervical

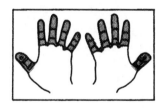

Look at the fingers. Observe the visual cues. Are the fingers straight? Crooked? How crooked? Curled when the hand is at rest? How curled? Which fingers? Are there wear spots on the fingers? Which fingers? Is

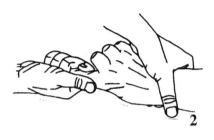

2

there callousing? Where? How much? On both hands? Are the fingers puffy? Are the fingernails regularly shaped? Irregularly shaped? Are they brittle and split? Do any show signs of injury such as irregular shape or a partial nail? What color are the nails? Pink/white? Yellow? Bluish? Pure white? Are all uniform in color? Do any or all show vertical ridges? Horizontal ridges? Spots of white? Small black splinter-like areas underneath?

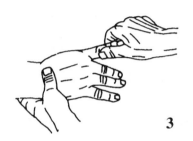

3

(2) Apply the pull technique to each of the fingers. Does the individual report pain, discomfort or feelings of stress in response?

(3) Apply the walk down/pull against technique to each of the fingers, both the tops of the fingers and the lateral aspects. Observe the degree of stretch possible when technique is applied to each of the individual's digits. Are the digits and joints uniform in degree of stretch? If not, which are unique? Do these digits or joints show signs of visual stress cues? Does the individual comment about sensitivity during the stretch? Does the joint show signs of visual stress cues?

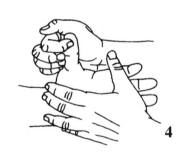

4

(4) Apply the modified grip technique to the pituitary / hypothalamus reflex area. Is it sensitive? How sensitive? What do you feel?

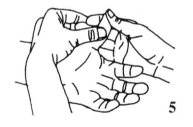

5

(5) Apply the thumb walking technique to the thumb. Note touch cues around the joints. Is there sensitivity? Do you feel hard tonus?

(6) Apply the thumb walking technique to the thyroid / parathyroid / neck / throat reflex area. Is there sensitivity? What do you feel? Thickness? Stringiness? Thumb walk across the area from the opposite direction. What do you feel?

(**7**) Apply the thumb walking technique to each of fingers. Consider the touch cues. What do you feel? Puffiness? Thickness? Hard tonus? Stringiness? Where? Consistently in all fingers?

(**8**) Apply the thumb walking technique to walk up the fingers. What do you feel? How do stress cues compare to those observed previously?

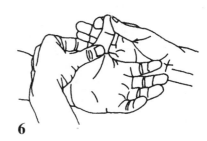

6

(**9**) Apply the side to side movement technique to each of the fingers. Observe the degree of movement possible when technique is applied to each of the individual's digits. Are the digits and joints uniform in degree of movement? If not, which are unique? Do these digits or joints show signs of visual stress cues? Is noise produced when any of the joints is moved? Which one(s)? Does the joint show signs of visual stress cues? Does the individual comment on the sound or comment about sensitivity during movement?

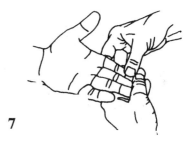

7

Consider the overall picture you have observed in the fingers. Have you noted multiple stress cues? In the thumb? In all the fingers? Were the observed stress cues also sensitive to pressure technique application? Do you consider the fingers to show signs of alarm, adaptation, or exhaustion? Do you consider the stress cues to be local, regional, or general in nature? Are there a sufficient number of stress cues to prompt you to ask the individual about his or her perception of stress in a corresponding body part? Note the overall stress pattern and keep it in mind as you work through the hand.

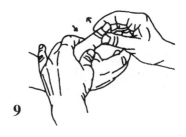

9

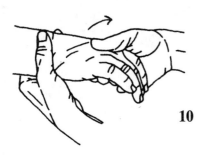

10

(10) Move the hand into an abducted position. Hold for several seconds. Did the hand move easily? **(11)** Move the hand into an adducted position. Hold for several seconds. Did the hand move easily?

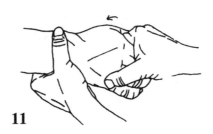

11

Thenar eminence

Right hand / Left hand

adrenal gland / adrenal gland

stomach (part) / stomach

pancreas (part) / pancreas

midback/spine / midback/spine

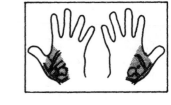

Observe the thenar eminence of the hand for visual stress cues. Is there thickness? Puffiness? Where? **(12)** Apply the modified grip technique to the adrenal reflex area. What do you feel? Does the individual respond with a report of sensitivity? How sensitive?

12

(13) Apply the thumb walking technique to the thenar eminence in a pattern of successive passes. What do you feel? Thickness? Lack of tonus? Hard tonus? Stringiness? Where? Over how large an area? Is there a shape to the observed tonus?

13

(14) Apply the thumb walking technique in another pass. Does your picture of what you feel change?

This area of the hand includes a long list of reflex areas with many possibilities for stress cues. Observing the touch stress cues takes practice. Use the above list of reflex areas as a checklist for the site of possible touch stress cues.

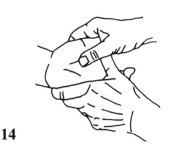

14

Consider the overall picture you have observed in the thenar eminence. Have you noted multiple stress cues? Were the observed stress cues also sensitive to pressure technique application? Do you consider the thenar eminence to show signs of alarm, adaptation, or exhaustion? Do you consider the stress cues to be local, regional, or general in nature? Are there a sufficient number of stress cues to prompt you to ask the individual about his or her perception of stress in a corresponding body part? Note the overall stress pattern and keep it in mind as you work through the hand. Compare the stress pattern in the thenar eminence to that of the fingers.

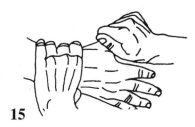

15

(15) Apply the pull technique to the thumb and each finger. (16) Apply the metacarpal grasp technique to each paired metacarpal heads. Did the hand move somewhat? easily? Barely?

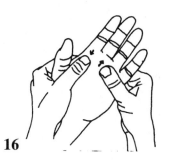

16

Ball of the hand

chest / lung / heart / breast

shoulder

upper back / between the shoulders

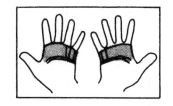

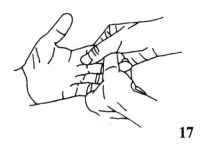

Observe the ball of the hand for visual stress cues. What is your overall impression? Is there callousing? Where? How thick? Over how large an area?

(17) Apply the thumb walking technique to the ball of the hand. What touch cues do you note? Is there sensitivity? Where? What do you feel? Is there thickening? Thickness? Lack of tonus? Hard tonus? Stringiness? Puffiness? Where? Over how large an area?

17

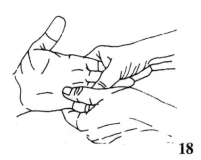

(18) Change working hands and apply the thumb walking technique to the shoulder area. Is there sensitivity? Thickness? Lack of tonus? Hard tonus?

Consider the stress cues you have observed in the hand thus far. Are there multiple stress cues in each of the fingers, the thenar eminence, and the ball of the hand? Is there an overall pattern of stress or a localized one? What reflex area observations have you made?

18

Body of the hand

Right hand / Left hand

solar plexus, diaphragm

liver/gallbladder / stomach/ spleen

upper back

arm/elbow

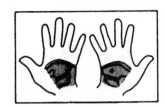

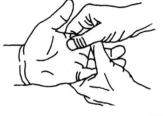

Observe the body of the hand for visual cues. Note any callousing, puffiness, or thickness. **(19)** Apply the thumb walking technique beginning with the solar plexus/diaphragm area and into the body of the hand. Is the area sensitive to pressure? Light pressure? Moderate

19

pressure? What do you feel? A stringy or thickened band? General thickness? What do you feel in the body of the hand? Stringiness? Thickness? Hard tonus? Is there shape to what you feel? (**20**) Change working hands and apply the thumb walking technique. What do you feel?

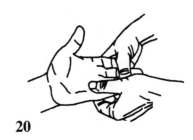

20

Consider the stress cues you have observed in the hand thus far. Are there multiple stress cues in any of the fingers, the ball of the hand, and the body? Is there an overall pattern of stress, a regional one, or a localized one? What reflex area observations have you made?

Heel

colon / colon

small intestine / small intestine

lower back/hip/pelvis / lower back/hip/pelvis

ileocecal valve / sigmoid colon

Observe the heel of the hand for visual stress cues. Is there callousing? White speckling? Where?

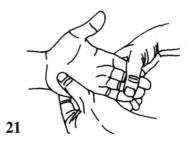

21

(**21**) Apply the thumb walking technique to the heel of the hand. Is there sensitivity? Thickness? Hard tonus? Do you feel a shape to the tonus? Note tonus and sensitivity in ileocecal valve and sigmoid areas.

(**22**) Apply the rotating on a point technique to the ovary/testicle reflex area. Is there sensitivity? What do you feel?

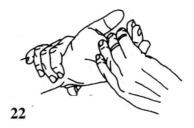

22

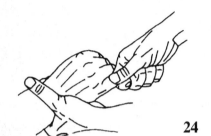

23

(23) Apply the rotating on a point technique to the uterus/prostate reflex area. Is there sensitivity? What do you feel?

(24) Apply the pull technique to the thumb and each finger.

(25) Apply the metacarpal mover technique. Does the hand move easily? Somewhat? Barely?

Once again, consider the stress cues you have observed on the hand thus far.

24

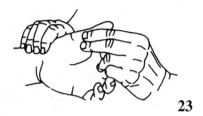

25

Hand Held in a Vertical Position

Inside of the hand

spine

tailbone

bladder

rectum

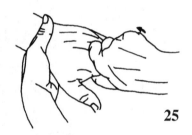

26

Observe the hand for visual stress cues. Is there puffiness? Callousing? Where? **(26)** Apply the thumb walking technique to the outer edge of the first metacarpal. Is there sensitivity? Where? What do you feel? Where? Puffiness? Thickness? Hard tonus?

Consider the stress cues you have observed in the hand to thus far. Have you observed an overall consistency to the stress cues?

Thenar eminence

Right hand / Left hand

heart

adrenal gland / adrenal gland

stomach (part) / stomach

pancreas (part) / pancreas

midback/spine / midback/spine

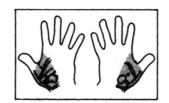

Recall the visual and touch stress cue observations noted in work on the thenar eminence with the hand held horizontally. **(27)** Apply the thumb walking technique in successive passes with the hand held vertically. Does your view of touch stress cues alter?

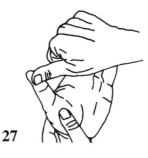

27

Webbing of the hand

between the shoulder blades

kidney / kidney

stomach

(28) Apply thumb walking or simultaneous thumb and finger walking to the webbing of the hand between the first and second metacarpals. Consider the touch stress cues. Do you feel thickness? Stringiness? Is there sensitivity? Where? Does the individual report tension between the shoulder blades? Do you observe stringiness in the area reported to be sensitive? Does the individual report a past injury to the upper back, collar bone or a rib?

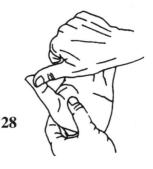

28

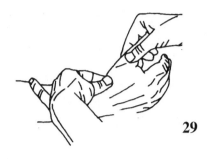

29

Is there an overall pattern of stress or one that is localized to an area or areas? Compare the stress cues you have observed in the webbings of the hand to those you observed in the ball of the hand. Are there multiple stress cues in both? Are both uniform in stress cue observations and stress inferences?

(**29**) Apply the metacarpal lever technique. Does the hand move easily? Somewhat? Barely?

Ball of the hand/webbings between fingers

chest / lung / heart / breast

solar plexus / diaphragm

shoulder

upper back / between the shoulders

eye / ear

tops of shoulders

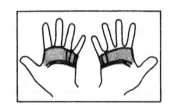

Recall the visual and touch stress cue observations noted in work on the ball of the hand with the hand held horizontally. (**30**) Apply the thumb walking technique in successive passes with the hand held vertically. Does your view of touch stress cues alter?

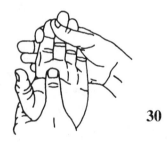

30

(**31**) As you apply thumb walking technique between the metacarpal heads, continue the thumb walking technique into the webbing between fingers, the eye / ear / tops of the shoulders reflex area. Consider the touch cues. Is there sensitivity? What does it feel like to you? Thickened tonus? Hard tonus? Stringiness?

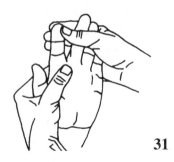

31

Where? Do you feel prompted to ask the client a question about an observed touch stress cue? If between the second and third fingers, does the individual report eye strain? Visual problems? If between the third and fourth fingers, does the individual report upper back tension or stress on tops of the shoulders? If between the fourth and fifth fingers, does the individual report hearing problems or ringing in the ears?

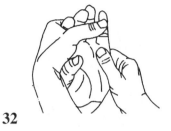

32

(**32**) Change working hands and apply thumb walking technique to the shoulder reflex area.

Body of the hand

Right hand / Left hand

upper back

arm/elbow

liver/gallbladder / stomach/ spleen

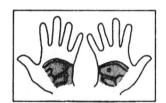

Recall the visual and touch stress cue observations noted in work in the body of the hand with the hand held horizontally. (**33**) Apply the thumb walking technique in successive passes with the hand held vertically. Does your view of touch stress cues alter from that noted previously? Do you feel stringiness, thickened tonus? Hard tonus?

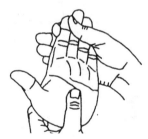

33

(**34**) Apply thumb walking or simultaneous thumb and finger walking to the fleshy outer edge of the hand. What do you feel? Is there sensitivity? How do these observations compare to your observations of the shoulder reflex area?

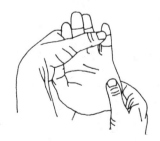

34

Heel

colon / colon

small intestine / small intestine

lower back/hip/pelvis / lower back/hip/pelvis

ileocecal valve / sigmoid colon

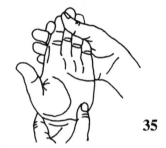

35

Recall the visual and touch stress cue observations noted in work on the heel with the hand held horizontally.

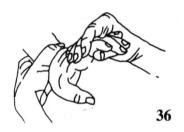

36

(35) Apply the thumb walking technique in successive passes with the hand held vertically. Does your view of touch stress cues alter?

Once again, consider the stress cues you have observed on the hand thus far.

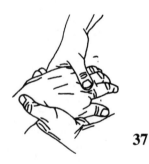

37

(36) Move the hand into a position of extension. Hold for several seconds. Does the hand stretch easily? Somewhat? Barely?

(37) Move the hand into a position of flexion. Hold for several seconds. Does the hand stretch easily? Somewhat? Barely?

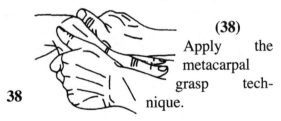

38

(38) Apply the metacarpal grasp technique.

Dorsal surface of the hand

head

neck

tops of shoulders

chest / breast

spine

lung / shoulder

upper back

hip / sciatic

knee / leg

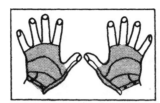

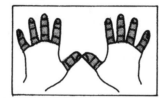

Observe the top of the hand for visual stress cues. Note the fingernails. **(39)** Apply the thumb walking technique to the spine reflex area of the first metacarpal.

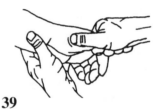

39

(40) Apply the thumb walking technique to the body of the hand. Is there sensitivity? Hard tonus? Stringiness? Where?

40

(41) Make successive passes of thumb walking technique along and between the metacarpal bones.

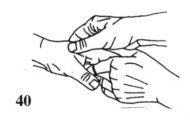

(42) Apply thumb walking technique to the arm/ shoulder reflex area. How do touch stress cues compare to previous work on the reflex area?

41

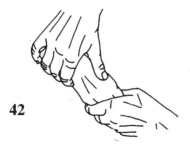

42

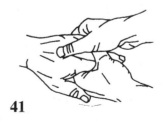

Wrist

ovary / testicle

uterus / prostate

fallopian tubes

lymphatic system

lower back / pelvis

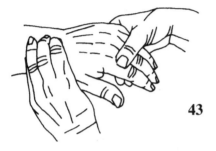

Observe the hand for visual stress cues. Is there puffiness? Thickness? **(43)** Apply the rotating on a point technique to the uterus/prostate reflex area.

43

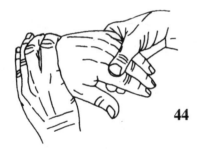

(44) Apply the rotating on a point technique to the ovary/testicle reflex area. How do sensitivity and touch stress cues compare to the reflex areas on the ventral surface?

44

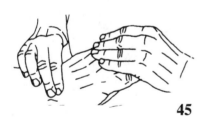

(45) Apply the finger walking technique to the dorsal surface of the carpal bones. Is there sensitivity? Thickness? Bumps of hard tonus?

(46) Apply the thumb walking technique to the tops of the fingers. Is there sensitivity? What do you feel? Thickness? Hard tonus especially around the joints?

(47) Apply the pull technique to the thumb and each finger.

45

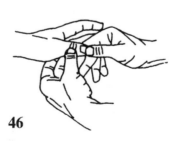

46

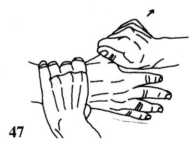

47

(48) Apply the walk down / pull against technique to each finger. Is there sensitivity? Does the finger move some?

(49) Apply the metacarpal grasp technique.

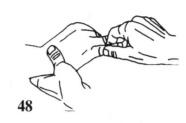

48

(50) Apply technique to the other hand, retracing items 1 through 49, and observing stress cues. As you work through the second hand, compare it to the first hand. Are the two hands about equal in stress cues? Does one show markedly more stress cues than the other? Where?

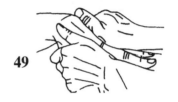

49

Summary

Consider the overall picture you have observed in the hand. Are there visual, touch, press and assess, and sensitivity cues about equal throughout the hand? Or do you note local, concentrated areas of stress cues? Have you observed a region of the hand, such as the fingers, that shows more stress cues than the others? Is there a general pattern of stress cues throughout the hand such as within the musculo-skeletal system? Do you note a general lack of stress cues? Do you consider there to be signs of alarm, adaptation, or exhaustion? Do you consider the stress cues to be local, regional, or general in nature? Are there a sufficient number of stress cues to prompt you to ask the individual about his or her perception of stress in a corresponding body part?

As you work through the second hand, compare it to the other hand. Are the two hands about equal in stress cues? Does one show markedly more stress cues than the other?

Reading the Hand: Stress Assessment

To read the hand (1) Select a part of the hand, such as the finger, for assessment. (2) Review the reflex areas in that part of the hand. (3) Determine whether or not there are any hand stress cues associated with the reflex area. (4) Consider the comments made by the individual about his or her response to stress.

This chart should be used only as a guide and not as a diagnostic tool.

Hand Part	Summary Chart		
	Hand Stress Cue	**Reflex Stress Inference**	**Body Stress Response**
Finger (**Distal phalanx**)	Puffiness, thickness, hard tonus	Head / brain / sinus	Headaches, sinus problems
Interphalangeal joint (**between distal and middle phalanges**)	Thickness / lacking tonus / hard tonus, sensitivity		Sinusitis, sinus headaches, neck problems
Middle Phalanx	Stringiness, thickness	Neck	Neck tension to neck problems
	Sensitivity, puffiness to thickness	Throat	Sore throat
	Sensitivity, thickened to stringy tonus	Thyroid / parathyroid	Low energy
Interphalangeal joint (**between middle and proximal phalanges**)	Thickness to hard tonus	Teeth / gum / jaws	Jaw injury / problems, dental problems

Hand Part	Summary Chart		
	Hand Stress Cue	**Reflex Stress Inference**	**Body Stress Response**
Webbing between fingers	Thickening to thickened to hard tonus, stringiness	Tops of shoulders	Tension in the tops of the shoulders, shoulder
(between second and third fingers)	Sensitivity, thickening to thickened to hard tonus	Eyes	Eye strain
(between second and third fingers)	Thickened to hardened tonus, sensitivity	Eyes	Eye problems
(between third and fourth fingers)	Sensitivity, thickening tonus	Ear	Ringing in the ears
(between third and fourth fingers)	Hard tonus, sensitivity	Ear	Hearing or ear problems
(between second and third fingers)	Hard tonus, sensitivity	Inner ear	Dizziness (such as when rising from a chair), vertigo, balance
Webbing of hand	Thickness, stringiness, lacking tonus	Between the shoulder blades, clavicle, ribs	Upper back problems, shoulder tension or problems
Ball of hand	Visual puffiness, thickened to hard to stringy tonus, sensitivity	Solar plexus	General tension, emotional response, breathing

Hand Part	Summary Chart		
	Hand Stress Cue	**Reflex Stress Inference**	**Body Stress Response**
	Speckled coloring to sheets of white / red, thickened to hardened tonus	Lungs	Frequent colds, lung problems
	Thickened to lacking to hardened tonus, sensitivity, puffiness	Chest / breast	Tension in the chest, breast problems
(fifth metacarpal head)	Thickening to thickened to lacking to hard tonus	Shoulder	Shoulder injury/problems
(first metacarpal head)	Puffiness to thickened to hardened tonus	Heart	Tension in the chest, heart problems
Thenar eminence	Sensitivity, thickened to hard tonus	Adrenal glands	Infection, asthma, allergies, hay fever, sinus problems/headaches, low energy
	Puffy to thickened tonus, visual puffiness, sensitivity	Pancreas	Low energy, highs and lows of energy, emotional stress
	Callousing or visual puffiness, sensitivity, puffy to thickened to hard tonus	Kidney	Kidney problems, mid to lower back problems

Hand Part	Summary Chart		
	Hand Stress Cue	**Reflex Stress Inference**	**Body Stress Response**
	Visual puffiness/ thickening, thickened to hard tonus, sensitivity	Stomach	Stomach problems, tension in the stomach
Body of hand	Stringy to thickened to hard tonus, sensitivity	Gallbladder	Digestive problems, flatulence
	Thickening to hard tonus, sensitivity	Large intestine	Digestive problems, foot/knee/hip joint problems
	Thickened to hard tonus, sensitivity	Liver	Digestive problems, immune response problems
	Stringy to thickened to hard tonus, sensitivity	Spleen	Anemia, immune response problems
	Speckled coloring to sheets of white/ red, thickened to lacking, to hard tonus, callousing	Upper back	Upper back tension/problems, whiplash
	Callousing, lacking to thickened to hard tonus, sensitivity	Arm / elbow	Arm problems such as weakness or aching, elbow, shoulder, or neck problems

Hand Part	Summary Chart		
	Hand Stress Cue	**Reflex Stress Inference**	**Body Stress Response**
Heel	Thickened to lacking to hard tonus, sensitivity	Colon, lower back, hip, pelvis, reproductive organs	Digestive problems, lower back problems, reproductive problems
	Thickening to lacking to hard tonus	Small intestine	Digestive problems
Inside of hand	Puffiness, sensitivity, thickened to hard tonus	Rectum	Digestive problems, hemorrhoids
	Sensitivity, puffy to thickened to hard tonus, bump, visible speckling or other color	Spine	Injury, back tension /problems, digestive problems, reproductive problems
	Puffiness, sensitivity, thickened to hard tonus	Bladder / lower back	Bladder problems, lower back problems
Outside of hand	Sensitivity, puffiness to lacking to thickened tonus	Knee / leg	Knee / leg problems
	Thickened to hard tonus, sensitivity	Arm, elbow, knee	Digestive problems, arm, elbow or knee problems
Top of hand (fingers)	Coloration of fingernail, misshapen fingernails		

Hand Part	Summary Chart		
	Hand Stress Cue	**Reflex Stress Inference**	**Body Stress Response**
	Knobby joints	Neck	Neck problems
Top of hand (body of hand)	Taut tendons	Upper back	Upper back tension
	Sensitivity, puffy to thickened to hard tonus	Lower back, hip/ sciatic	Lower back tension /problems, sciatic problems
Wrist	Visual puffiness/ thickness, puffy to thickened tonus, hard tonus	Lymphatic glands, fallopian tubes, groin, lower back	Wrist injury / swelling, reproductive problems, wrist problems, lower back problems
	Visual puffiness, sensitivity, thickened to hard tonus	Uterus / prostate	Reproductive problems

CHAPTER 12

The Session

Putting the techniques together into a coherent pattern is in itself an important part of reflexology. The goal of the session is to combine application of technique, assessment of stress cues, and consideration of the individual into an organized, consistent approach to get results and to create a relaxing experience. This requires the balancing of sufficient technique application to create change in the stress mechanism within the individual's ability to respond to technique application.

The integrated hand reflexology session causes a relaxation response because it provides an appropriate level of pressure technique application. Each individual comes to you with a pre-set level of stress adaptation and predetermined goals for a session. Effectively and efficiently creating a relaxation response involves consideration of technique application during a session and over a series of sessions. The goal of this chapter is to describe to you aspects of successful session planning.

The session pattern is a systematic, repeatable method of applying technique to the hand. It affords you an opportunity to assess the hand in a systematic manner. Technique specifically tailored to the individual is then applied. The session includes: (1) working through a hand once to apply pressure technique to the entire hand and to observe stress cues on the entire hand and (2) working through the hand a second time, applying pressure technique to areas of emphasis (stress cues) selected during the first work through.

Going through the hand systematically is a way of organizing a plan of action. It gives you an opportunity to gather your thoughts about the stress patterns, to create priorities for further technique application, and to seek information that clarifies the individual's stress pattern. Technique is applied to the entire hand at least once to contribute to the goal of relaxing the entire body and its stress mechanism.

Going through the hand a second time allows you to emphasize technique application appropriate to the individual's stress pattern. The individual's stress pattern may consist of a hand stress pattern, a reflex stress pattern, a body stress pattern, or any combination of the three. You want to match your technique application to the individual's stress pattern to produce optimal results. The skill you develop is the ability to customize your technique application to that individual. The science of reflexology may be the application of pressure technique, but the art of reflexology is in your response to the individual as a whole.

The four-stage process described in this chapter is designed to guide you through the elements of a session. Providing a session is the application of technique appropriate to relax the stresses of a particular individual. The goal of the session is to (1) Apply technique to the hands with a strategy appropriate to the stress cue inferences; (2) Interview the individual to gather information about his or her stress history, relaxation goals, and expectations; (3) Develop a session strategy that best provides relaxation for that individual; (4) Document the strategy to form a reflexological stress assessment and plan of future work within a standard medical format.

Applying Technique to the Hand

Pressure triggers the body's ability to return to a less stressed state. Pressure technique strategy is selected for its appropriateness in interrupting, conditioning, and educating the hand. Every pair of hands is a puzzle with the question, "How can this hand best be unlocked from its pattern of stress?"

Philosophy of Technique Application to Relax Stress

Stress researcher Hans Selye noted the stereotypical response of the body to stress as a progression through the stages of alarm, adaptation, and exhaustion. The reflexologist assesses the hand and notes the stages of adaptation. The reflexologist then elicits a relaxation response by applying a consistent program of pressure to the hands. The stereotypical response of the body to such pressure application is a progression through the stages of interruption, conditioning, and education. The stimulus of pressure interrupts stress and evokes a response of relaxation. Pressure technique applied consistently over time creates a conditioned, reflexive response. Such technique application interferes with the stress pattern on a frequency basis sufficient to create change. Continued technique application is an educational exercise within brain-organ dynamics.

The technique that is just right lulls the hand and body into a sense of relaxation. The right level of pressure unlocks tissues, relaxes muscles, and causes change. The goal is to balance technique application with the hand's state of stress adaptation, alarm, adaptation, or exhaustion.
It is possible for pressure technique application to be insufficient to interrupt the stress mechanism. Heavily adapted

stressed areas of the hand tend to resist weak signals or light pressure. Heavily adapted areas also require a sophisticated approach to unlock the Rubik's cube of stress.

The signal of pressure itself is a stressor. It changes from being a good stressor to being a bad stressor when it is applied beyond the ability of the individual's stage of adaptation to cope with its application. For example, too much pressure applied to the already exhausted hands of an individual may cause further exhaustion. The art of reflexology is to remain under the person's range of tolerance, not above it.

Creating Change With Technique Application

The reflexologist applies pressure techniques to the hands for the purpose of interrupting the individual's stress pattern. This is accomplished by matching the appropriate technique application with the particular area of emphasis on the hand. The overall goal is a pattern of technique application to stressed areas on the hand that results in a change in overall stress patterns.

In applying technique to the hand, first consider the response of the hand to pressure technique. An initial application of technique interrupts the pattern of stress. Technique application over several sessions conditions the hand and creates a change in overall stress pattern. Ongoing work educates the hand to respond to stress in the best possible manner.

Next, consider the individual's initial pattern of stress adaptation. The rate at which a change in stress patterns takes place varies according to the individual's initial stress pattern – whether it is alarm, adaptation, or exhaustion. Remember the Basic Rule of hand Stress / Relaxation: The more the adaptation to stress over the longer the period of time: (1) The more pronounced the stress cue. (2) The more deeply ingrained the pattern of stress. (3) The greater the potential for the individual's awareness of stress and/or stress-related problems. (4) The more conditioning by pressure technique application will be required over a longer period of time to change the pattern of stress.

To change a pattern of stress from any one stage of adaptation to another requires consistent, systematic technique application, including where to apply technique, how much pressure to apply, how many passes to make, and how many sessions are suggested. Your goal with technique strategy is to achieve the maximum effect with a minimum of effort. The most effective application of technique provides an appropriate level of challenge.

Technique Strategy

How much pressure to use, how frequently to apply that pressure, where to apply pressure, and how many sessions will be required are questions asked by the reflexologist in determining a technique procedure that will most efficiently and effectively relax and condition the hand. Consider the application of pressure technique to be an opportunity to shape up and exercise the hand. Just as any exercise program provides guidelines for working with the body, the reflexologist utilizes a strategy of exercise procedures to appropriately condition the hand.

Consider the evaluation of the hand discussed in the previous chapter. The local, regional, and general patterns of stress encountered on a hand are measured according to alarm, adaptation, and exhaustion stages. The technique strategy you use to elicit a relaxation response will be matched to the patterns of stress adaptation. Pressure is your working tool. The amount of pressure, the number of passes, and the number of sessions reflect the reflexologist's answers to the basic questions of how much pressure to apply, how long to apply it, and where to apply it.

Technique Strategy: How Much Pressure to Apply

The reflexologist works with a "variable speed" thumb walking technique, with the ability to provide a variety of pressure levels from light to medium to heavy to any number of gradations in between. Observe the hand. Consider the cues that you see and feel. Work for change in the area of the hand to which you are applying technique. Work within the comfort zone of the individual. Practice applying a variety of pressure levels to an area of the hand and note the response of each.

Light Pressure

Light pressure is a level of pressure that interrupts stress and does not challenge it. Stress cues of exhaustion and extreme sensitivity, the hand of an older person, or an infant's hand call for a light touch. In addition, light pressure is a "warm-up" level of pressure for applying thumb walking technique. When starting work on a hand, you are testing to see what level of pressure is appropriate, in general, for the individual's hand. Start lightly and adjust pressure according to the response you get. Some hands will respond only to light pressure throughout the session.

Light pressure in itself can be utilized purely as a relaxation technique. Light pressure application can also provide a quick evaluation of the hand to generally gauge touch stress cues in an area, region, or the whole hand.

Medium Pressure

Medium pressure describes a moderate level of challenge used with a hand that shows signs of the adaptation stage. A lack of visual stress cues, a general consistent thickness throughout the hand, and/or moderate sensitivity to technique application call for a level of technique application that challenges the hand moderately. It is a level of pressure that you will find works effectively with almost anyone, and it is the level of pressure you will be working with most of the time. "It hurts good" is a comment frequently heard in reference to this level of pressure.

Heavy Pressure

Heavy pressure describes an upper range of challenge utilized for the highly adapted hand. Callousing or thick, heavy hands with no sensitivity or hands that have been conditioned by the application of moderate pressure over time call for technique application of a sufficient magnitude to cause a response. Heavy pressure may be appropriate when medium pressure does not seem to bring a response.

Heavy pressure is not a beginning level pressure. It is not appropriate for all individuals. However, some individuals prefer a more vigorous work- out and they may request more pressure. For these individuals, a heavy level of pressure "hurts good."

Take care not to overstress your own thumb. The leverage of the working hand is particularly important in applying this level of pressure. Also, be aware of the effect your technique application has on the individual. Sensitivity levels will change during the course of a session. You may find a sudden breakthrough where a previously insensitive area is suddenly sensitive.

Technique Strategy: Frequency of Passes

The frequency of passes of pressure techniques over a particular area is gauged by the amount of pressure you are using. The lighter the pressure, the more frequent the passes needed to achieve a conditioning effect.

5 to 10 Passes: Five to ten passes of thumb walking technique are sufficient to assess an area for stress cues or to apply medium or heavy pressure.

10 to 15 Passes: By applying ten to fifteen passes you are condi-

tioning the hand with light to medium pressure.

15 to 20 Passes: Fifteen or more passes show special attention to a stressed area that calls for light pressure. If you are applying 15 to 20 passes of medium to heavy pressure, consider other technique strategies. (See below.)

Technique Strategy: Where to Apply Technique

Strategy One: Approach

The technique strategy you use to elicit a relaxation response will be matched to the patterns of stress adaptation. Pressure is your working tool and the stress cue is your target for where to apply technique. The evaluation of the hand discussed in the previous chapter provides you with an evaluation of each stress cue. A stress cue such as puffiness should be approached with technique application appropriate to an alarm stage of adaptation.

Approach is also a technique procedure for noting what the individual likes. Techniques and parts of the hand to which the individual responds favorably should be emphasized. When the individual comments "That feels good," note the technique you are using and/or the part of the hand being worked. The area can be used as the individual's relaxation area, somewhat akin to the solar plexus area – as an overall area of relaxation. This individual is responding to your work. It may just feel good to the individual or it may be an indicator of a key area or technique likely to cause a change in a stress pattern and/or mechanism.

Strategy Two: Avoidance

Avoidance is a technique procedure for noting parts of the hand to which pressure should **not** be applied. Cuts, bruises, and any injured part of the hand signal a part of the hand to be avoided.

Avoidance is also a technique procedure for noting the technique or parts of the hand to which the individual responds negatively. Most frequently this will be a response of extreme sensitivity. The individual reports that "It hurts bad" or "The technique you are applying is bothering me." It may be a transitory feeling or it may be an indicator of a key area or technique likely to cause distress. In any event, indicate that you will avoid working on the area or applying the technique until such time that the hand is conditioned to the point that further work is possible. Consider the possible causes of their response. Focus on the area as a stress cue of extreme sensitivity that requires further observation. Listen to what the individual says about a possible source of his or her response. In addition, if technique application causes pain that persists beyond the session or if a part of the hand feels bruised to the touch following technique application, the area has been overworked. Reevaluate the area and consider another approach.

Strategy Three: Working the Surrounding Area

Working the surrounding area is a technique strategy utilized to work with the stress cue that is resistant to change or that is to be avoided. Stress cues such as extreme sensitivity, sensitivity that increases rather than decreases with work, corns, and callousing are typical areas that can be better approached indirectly. To apply the technique procedure, apply technique to the area adjacent to the area of sensitivity, gradually working closer and closer to the area of interest. When appropriate, apply thumb walking technique directly to the area of interest to test for change in the stress cue such as sensitivity. Consider also approaching the stress cue by way of "Systems" or "Zones."

Working the surrounding area is also utilized rather than repeatedly applying thumb walking technique to a stressed area. It provides a break in technique application to an area of interest and allows time for the hand to adapt and create a change in the stress pattern.

Strategy Four: Working From Several Directions

The goal of this technique procedure is to gather more information and to provide variety to the stressed area. Once a part of the hand has drawn your attention through observation of a stress cue, approach the area of interest from several viewpoints. Thumb walking technique applied from several different directions provides a depth to your assessment and technique application. The stress cue may be apparent from one directional approach but not another. Sensitivity may be elicited from working one direction and not another. The individual may even report that one particular directional approach feels "good" and thus better than other approaches.

Strategy Five: Note Any Change

To consider the effect of your work, note any change that takes place in response to your pressure technique application. Consider the area under your thumb after a few passes. Consider a region of the hand after some work. Finally, consider the whole hand after technique application. Note any change in size, shape, or dimensions of the stress cue in response to your work. Note any shift in sensitivity response. **Remember the Basic Rule of Change within the Stress Pattern. The more quickly change occurs in response to pressure, the less the impact of the stress, the shorter the duration of time it has been there, and the less time required to condition the hand**.

Strategy Six: Self-help

Self-help techniques are technique procedures applied by the client between sessions. The value of self-help is twofold: It encourages individuals to get involved in their own health, and it speeds up results. Your client may or may not be interested in learning everything about reflexology or the techniques, but he or she may be interested in an appropriate self-help technique or two. Choose your objectives. Target only a limited number of areas for your client to work on, because self-help homework can be confusing and unusable if not clearly and simply defined. For further information, see Kunz and Kunz, *Hand And Hand Reflexology, A Self-Help Guide*, New York, Simon & Schuster, 1984.

Technique Strategy: Number of Sessions

How many sessions of pressure technique application will be required to cause a conditioning effect? Remember, the stimulus of pressure interrupts stress and evokes a response of relaxation. Pressure technique applied consistently over time creates a conditioning effect. The actual number of sessions necessary to achieve a goal varies from individual to individual; however, the number of sessions necessary to cause a conditioning effect is predictable.

Interrupting Stress Response

The goal of interrupting stress takes place during any one session. Most individuals experience a feeling of relaxation all over the body. The individual who does not experience a relaxation effect immediately will require three to five sessions to break the established pattern of stress. Many individuals report a change in their perception of their hands. They will often state that they didn't realize their hands could feel so relaxed, that their hands feel lighter, or that they feel their hands are less stiff.

Conditioning Stress Response

A conditioning effect should take place with subsequent sessions once or twice a week over a two to four week period. The individual should report that the relaxation effect spans a progressively longer time period. Change has taken place when the individual reports alarm-level stress cues that are less sensitive and adapted cues that show change. Some ongoing technique application will be needed to maintain the conditioning effect. A session every two weeks or once a month with some self-help should maintain the level of conditioning.

Educating Stress Response

With four to eight weeks of technique application, the individual should report a more lasting effect. Education has taken place when little or no sensitivity is reported and many of the adapted stress cues show change. On-going technique application every two weeks or once a month with self-help will maintain and up-keep the conditioning effect.

Variables

A very ill person may respond immediately to technique application. Any lessening of the individual's stressed and exhausted state can create dramatic contrast. Ironically, less technique application may be required to create a change with the very sick or chronically ill individual.

Consider it a "stubborn" stress response when the individual reports little change from session to session. This individual may have a hard time relaxing and may be conditioned to an overall high tension level. More technique application is needed over a longer period of time to condition and create a change. (Make it a goal to reduce the overall stress level. Consider a session with multiple desserts and light pressure applied to the solar plexus reflex area and the individual's key stress cues.)

Interviewing the Individual

The interchange with the individual is an important part of any session. In talking to the owner of the hand before, during, and after your session, you are gathering more information, giving an assessment to the individual, and, overall, demonstrating your professional competence. The interview is a focused, systematic effort to communicate your findings and to elicit the individual's feelings.

Some individuals will immediately tell you what you need to know about their stress level. This individual will comment on his or her stress history, goals for your work with him or her, and his or her perception of your work as it progresses. Other individuals will need prompting to describe their feelings. Either way, you will want a consistent, systematic method to interview the individual. The interview during the session tells you what stress factors and relaxation goals are present. This information combined with your findings will determine how much conditioning and what type will be required to relax the individual's stress pattern.

The interview includes listening, asking questions, and being observant of verbal cues. You want to get the person talking. Asking questions focuses the individual on his or her stress pattern and goals. In addition, a systematic interview focuses your work on developing a session custom tailored for that individual.

Stress History

The individual's hands in front of you are a history of who the individual is, what he or she has been doing, and how long he or she has been doing it. To respond with a session that is right for the individual, the reflexologist considers the individual's preset level of tension. The starting point for your work is, in essence, the individual's overall level of background tension. The preset tension level includes the exposure of the individual's hand and body to use, overuse, illness, and/or injury.

Time is a factor that indicates how long a particular stress has affected the individual. How old is the individual? How much time has he or she spent or is spending at a standing, sitting, stressful, or physical occupation? How many injuries, car accidents, major illnesses, and so forth has the individual experienced and at what age? How long has it been since an injury or stressful event occurred? This information is important to the reflexologist in planning his or her session. Remember, the longer something has been adapted to, the greater the possibility that it has become established as a stress pattern. It follows that the more serious the stress event and/or the more stress events or injuries at a younger age, the more complex the stress pattern.

The stress history portion of the interview allows you to note the impact of past and current stress by gathering information about age, occupation, and stress events. **The Basic Rule of a Stress History is (1) The older the individual, (2) the longer the time since the stress event, (3) the greater the impact of the stress or stress event, and (4) the more time spent in a sitting or standing or walking occupation or physical occupation the greater the chance for ingrained wear-and-tear patterns and injury and the more technique application will be required to interrupt, condition, or educate the stress mechanism.**

Age

Selye considered the stages of adaptation to be analogous with the stages of life. Childhood compared to the alarm stage because of the learning aspects of both; adult ages paralleled the adaptation stage; older ages compared to the exhaustion phase of adaptation.

Children and young adults are still growing. Because children's bodies have yet to fully establish a response to stress, patterns of stress are not deeply ingrained. Thus, you can expect to observe lesser stress cues, sharp areas that respond quickly to technique application, and, in general, quicker changes than are observable in an adult.

The older the person, obviously, the greater the potential for deeply ingrained stress patterns, as there is a greater potential for past stress events such as injury. In general, it may be more difficult to interrupt stress and to maintain the interruption. In turn, the more stress cues you observe and the older the individual, the less aggressive the approach you should take. Applying challenging techniques to an exhausted hand may elicit more exhaustion.

Occupation and Hobby

Work (e.g., computer-user, construction worker, factory worker) creates particular stresses for the hand and body. Signs of hand overuse and adaptation are common in many occupations. The longer the workday and the more years on the hands, the greater the potential for fatigue throughout the hand. Additional stresses can be created by working in a fixed position. In addition, physical occupations such as construction and assembly work offer the potential for injury and overuse. The hand shows signs of adaptation and fatigue.

Hobbies also provide the potential for hand stress and injury. Most sports activities include the use of the hand to grip (e. g., tennis, golf, bowling), to catch (e.g., basketball, football) or to compete in general. The possibilities of over-use and injury are many. Even hobbies such as computer game playing, musical and craft activities contain the potential for the stress of overuse of the hands (e.g., the wear and tear on the finger joints and following hours of holding a computer game, guitar playing, crocheting).

Stress

To get an idea about the individual's perception of his or her health and stress level, ask a neutral question such as, "Are you in pretty good health?" Such a question will usually elicit a response that indicates whether the person perceives his or her body to be under stress and in what manner.

Asking a question such as, "Do you take pretty good care of yourself?" tells you how the person copes with stress. Such a question will typically elicit information about activities such as seeking medical help regularly, visiting the health spa frequently, taking vitamins, paying attention to diet and health habits, working out at home, or visiting a massage therapist, acupuncturist, or other therapist.

Stress Event

In response to a stress cue of note, a question such as, "Have you ever injured yourself?" will tell you how much stress the individual faces due to past stress events. Trauma to the body, especially the foot, is reflected as a stress experience observable on the hand. Take note of the report of any stress events such as a car accident, an operation, a high school sports-related injury, a major illness, or an on-the-job injury. How serious was the event and how long ago did it happen? Answers to these two questions provide a picture of how ingrained the stress adaptation has become.

In response to a stress cue of note, especially in the solar plexus reflex area, you might also ask, "Do you feel as if you are under stress?" Frequently the individual will respond with a report about stress at home or at the workplace.

Stress History and the Reflex Relaxation Scale

The existing stress patterns have an impact on how long it will take to create change. Age tells you how long the individual has accumulated the stress patterns. Stress events tell you what reflex patterns have been set up in response to accidents, injuries, and emotional distress.

In asking the question, "How long will it take to create change?" the learning curve in regard to conditioning reflexes is considered. Each stage of adaptation is evaluated in light of the stress history of the individual. When observing, for example, the hands of a young adult which show signs of exhaustion, consider the possibility that this person may have experienced a major stress event in his or her life. Thus, the amount of technique application to create change will be greater than that required for a young adult without the major stress event. The individual's stress history has a direct impact on their stage of adaptation. Stress history provides predictable elements that allow you to estimate the amount of technique application necessary to create a change in the reflex stress pattern.

Alarm: An alarm reflex pattern is not yet etched into the body's reflexive patterns. Children and individuals of any age with a recent injury, a recent stress, or a recent hand-use intensive occupation may be in this category.

Adaptation: Adult, or an individual of any age with a one to five year time period since injury, major stress, or in a hand-use intensive occupation.

Exhaustion: Older adult OR an individual of any age with a recent major injury, illness, operation, or stress, OR an individual with an injury or a stress that occurred five or more years ago, OR an individual in a hand-use intensive occupation for five or more years.

Eliciting Relaxation Goals

Most individuals have some sort of goal in mind when visiting a reflexologist. It is a part of the reflexologist's role to elicit and recognize goal statements from the individual. It is also a part of the reflexologist's role to consider whether or not the individual's expectations are realistic. These are skills developed by focusing on communication with the individual: listening, asking questions, and being observant in general to verbal cues.

At the start of a session, asking a question will give you a general idea of what the individual is seeking to accomplish through the use of reflexology. "What exactly are you looking for in reflexology?" or "Have you had your hands worked on before?" are questions that help create a focus for your session.

Consider the individual's response or general comment about goals. What, in general, is the individual signaling as a stress reduction goal? Is it a hand stress goal? Or is it a reflex stress goal? Is it a body goal or a combination of goals? Once the individual has indicated what part of the stress pattern he or she is interested in relaxing, consider the end result the person would like to see.

Typical comments or responses about stress patterns include:

Hand stress goals (tired hands): "My hands hurt." "I work with my hands all day." "I'm aware of the tension in my hands all the time."

Hand stress goals (hand problem, operation, injury): "I've had a hand operation, injury, and/or hand problem and I want to take better care of my hands." (*Note*: The reflexologist does not work with any hand problem that is undiagnosed.)

Reflex stress goal (stress-related condition, operation, injury): "My shoulder bothers me." "My digestion bothers me."

"I've heard reflexology could help with back problems." "My back bothers me all the time." "I've had surgery on my eyes." "I had a car accident six months ago." (*Note:* The reflexologist does not work with any undiagnosed or specific problem.)

Body stress goal (relaxation, stress reduction): "I've been stressed at home/work. I'm looking for anything to reduce my stress level."

Typical comments or responses about desired results include:

Prevention: "I'm interested in taking care of myself. I'd rather spend the money now to relax tension than later to pay medical bills."

Maintenance: "I like to do good things for my health."

Touch: "I'm single and I treat myself to these little luxuries."

Awareness: "I like having my hands worked on."

Performance: "I just don't feel that good any more." "I know I'm pushing my body, but I have deadlines to meet."

Matching Expectations

Now that the individual has told you his or her feelings and goals, consider your findings. A goal of relaxing tired hands, for example, is considered in relationship to the hand you are observing. How much stress is present in the hand and how much of a conditioning effect does the individual want to achieve? This will dictate the amount of technique application that will be required to reach the goal.

It is important to remember: (1) Some goals require more work than others; (2) Some goals are more ambitious than others; (3) Some goals require a shift in response to stress by the individual. What is realistically possible for the individual?

Any goal statement is a request for interruption of stress. Once you have applied technique and interrupted stress during a session, you would expect the individual to feel some relaxation of the stress. The individual, however, may also be seeking a longer lasting effect. Does the individual want his or her tired hands to feel better when walking out of your office after one session? Does the individual want his or her tired hands to feel better between sessions, for a week at a time? Or is the individual looking for a long-range solution to tired hands?

The skill comes from listening and considering what is possible for this individual with your session. It may not be easy to interrupt the stress pattern of, for example, a hand that is in the exhaustion stage of adaptation. It is important to match the individual's stage of adaptation with what can realistically be expected from the session. To match the individual's expectations with your findings, ask yourself, "What is the likely response to the application of technique?"

Interrupting stress: Is your expectation of the results of technique application that the individual will feel lessened stress after one session and that perhaps the feeling will last a few days?

Conditioning stress: Is your expectation of the results of technique application that the individual will feel lessened stress that will last between sessions, say a week or longer?

Educating stress: Is your expectation that the feeling of lessened stress will be continuous with some maintenance and that the individual may move on to some new goals?

Observing and Noting Changes in Stress Response

How do you know if you have reached your goal of creating a change in the individual's stress mechanism? Also, how does the individual know that he or she has received something of value through the application of reflexology technique?

Changes in tension level are observable. By observing and noting changes, the reflexologist provides himself or herself, as well as the client, with an opportunity to make an ongoing stress history to gauge response to technique application. Over the long term, progress toward the individual's goals can be measured. During the course of a session, you will observe and note changes in response to technique application, changes in the appearance of stress cues, in sensitivity, and in comments from the client.

Change in the hand stress mechanism is gauged by asking questions during the session. The answers will tell you how quickly and how much change took place in response to technique application. During the session, point out changes in the stress cues. For example, note, "This area is less puffy than it was." Or ask, "Is that area (a previously sensitive area, for example) as sensitive as it was?" "How does your hand feel?" "This area feels less pronounced to me. How does it feel to you?"

Note the individual's comments during the session. "My headache feels better." "I can't feel the tension between my shoulder blades any more." "I'm so relaxed I could fall asleep."

After work on one hand, ask the individual, "Would you mind flexing the fingers of your two hands? Now, do you feel a difference between the two hands?" The individual's response gives you feedback about how quickly he or she is responding (or is not responding) to your work. Answers range from "It feels like a new hand" to "It feels like a pillow" to "It's okay" to "It feels better than it did" to "It feels about the same."

At the finish of your work, asking, "How does that feel?" prompts the individual to note the effects of your work. Typical comments that gauge the response to the session include: "That feels better." (Indication that some interruption of stress has taken place.) "That feels great" or "That feels like a whole new hand." (Indication that interruption of stress has taken place.)

At the start of the next session ask, "How do you feel?" The individual will probably make a general response such as, "I feel pretty good" or "I feel about the same." A follow-up question to elicit more information is a statement and question such as "You felt pretty good at the end of the previous session. How long did that feeling last?" The individual's responses allow you to note any change in the overall stress mechanism. The individual who reports, "I felt good a few days after the last session" is signaling that, although stress was interrupted, the hand is not yet conditioned to a lesser stage of stress adaptation. The individual who reports, "I felt good the entire time between sessions" is signaling that conditioning has taken place. The individual who says, "I didn't even notice the stress condition this week" has reached an educated stage of adaptation. The level of response is a reflection of change in stress pattern following technique application.

With each session during the series, consider the ongoing progress of the stress pattern. Signs of a lasting improvement include, "I can type all day and my hands don't bother me any more" or "My hands feel like a million dollars" or "I suddenly realized I could turn my head in traffic without turning my whole body – my neck is doing so much better" or "I just plain feel better" or "I was under a lot of stress last week with work and I could handle it."

The Session Plan

Planning

Work with the client to create a plan of action to reduce his or her stress. A certain amount of technique application will be required to create the change he or she is seeking. To clarify the commitment necessary to achieve goals, discuss the amount of adaptation present and the amount of technique application required under the circumstances.

To match the individual's expectations with what you have observed on the hands, consider that the goal of reflexology is to provide relaxation and, over time, a conditioning effect. It is a basic tenet of reflexology that an adequate supply of technique application will cause a change in the stress mechanism. The more the adaptation to stress, the more the alteration of brain-organ dynamics and the more the application of technique required to create change.

The goal of the individual should be to apply pressure technique sufficient to teach the body a better adaptation to stress. The individual utilizes the services of the reflexologist and self-help as a tool to meet goals. Ask yourself if the individual has set realistic goals. For example, does the individual expect to reverse a lifetime of stress adaptations in one session? The reflexologist works to create a realistic goal by clarifying the amount of effort necessary to achieve the potential goal.

Give the individual a general evaluation of the stress and stress level you have observed in his or her hands. Include a general idea of your perspective of how much reflexology work would be appropriate and needed for his or her stress pattern. Your comments are framed in reference to the stage of adaptation and the wear-and-tear pattern you have observed. You give the individual an indication of his or her starting point stage of adaptation to suggest the extent of the technique application that will be required to cause a change. You want to apprise the individual about how much commitment will be needed on his or her part to reach the relaxation goal.

An example of such as approach is, "I see quite a few signs of adaptation (stress cues) that have been here for a while. The pattern of stress cues and your answers to questions seem to indicate that the pattern of stress has become a recurring problem to you. While you have experienced a few major stress events in the recent past, you have indicated that you have made an effort to take care of yourself. It will require regular technique application to achieve the goal of maintenance that you have indicated. I can do part of that and you can do part of that through self-help techniques."

Possible comments that can be used to signal your appraisal include:

Occasional stress "I see a few signs of stress. Your hands seem to be in pretty good overall shape. It shouldn't take a long time to condition these hands."

Recurring, moderate stress "I see a fair amount of stress cues but, overall, the hand seems to be in good shape. It will take a moderate amount of technique application to destress these hands. You can speed up the process and keep up with the stress level through self-help."

Chronic stress "I see quite a few stress cues that have been here for quite a while. It will take a while to condition these hands, but you can help speed the process with self–help."

The Session Procedure

The following is a step-by-step description of proceeding through a session. A systematic procedure allows you to concentrate your efforts on the individual because it frees you to emphasize technique application appropriate to that individual. Finally, an organized, consistent approach adds to your professional image.

Prepare your workplace. Wash your hands. Check your fingernail length. Check your workplace.

Begin your session. Invite the individual to sit and place his or her hand on the towel or pillow that forms the working surface.

Look over the entire hand for any area to be avoided. Ask the individual if there is any part of the hand that should be avoided, such as injured areas, cuts, bruises, rashes, infections, ingrown nails. Make sure any wound or break in the skin is covered. Look for the extreme stress cue that may indicate a part of the hand that should be approached carefully or avoided altogether.

Begin your technique application with a series of movement techniques to warm up the hand and, thus, prepare it for pressure technique application. A cold hand or a hand lacking in circulation may respond with more sensitivity. Make a preliminary assessment of visual stress cues. Consider your general impression of the hand, the most outstanding visual stress cues, and their locations.

Ask a general question about the individual's goals, such as, "Have you ever had your hands done before?" or "Are you familiar with reflexology?" or "Why did you decide to try reflexology?" At this point it may be necessary to clarify the nature of your service. If the individual is seeking medical services, note that you cannot treat for a specific illness. If the individual is experiencing an acute or undiagnosed problem, refer him or her to the appropriate medical services.

Consider what level of pressure is appropriate to begin your work. A thin adult hand, an older hand, a younger hand, or a hand very sensitive to initial contact call for a light touch. A heavy hand may require a heavy pressure to register a sensation.

Apply technique. As you work through the hands, adjust your pressure level by watching the individual's facial response to your work. To stay within the individual's comfort zone, ask the individual to tell you when the pressure of technique application is too much.

During the session, keep at least one hand on the hand on which you are working. In most cases this will be the holding hand because you will constantly be repositioning the working hand to work other areas. Your thumb or fingers may get tired. Learn how to vary your techniques to avoid fatigue. For example, when the walking thumb begins to tire, change to a movement technique, or switch hands and walk with the other thumb from the opposite direction. As you build your hand strength over a period of time, this will be less of a concern.

Follow a systematic, repeatable pattern to work through the hand. Make an assessment of the touch stress cues as you work. Consider the characteristics and location of the stress cues. Compare the stress cues in the fingers to those in the thenar eminence of the hand and other parts of the hand. Note sensitivity reported by the individual. Compare the touch cues to the visual cues. Gather information about the individual's perception of his or her stress.
After you work through the hand for the first time, consider your evaluation of the hand. Select areas of emphasis for technique application during the second time through the hand. Consider the pattern of technique application that would be most appropriate to relax the observed stress cues.

Work through the hand a second time, targeting selected areas of emphasis. Make a more detailed assessment of the areas of interest and the general pattern of stress. Note any change in the stress cue as technique is applied and after technique is applied. Consider whether any of the selected areas is more relaxed (i.e., a puffy area is less puffy, a thickened area is less thick). Apply a series of movement techniques to finish your work on the hand. Consider whether or not the hand feels more relaxed than it did during the initial series of movement techniques.

Ask the individual to flex the fingers on both hands to compare and contrast one hand with the other. Note the response to your work on the one hand.

Work through the other hand. Repeat the above procedures. Compare this hand to the first hand. Did you find similar stress cues? A similar overall feel to the hand? Widely different stress cues? More sensitivity?

At the end of the session, ask a question such as, "What do you think?" or "How do you feel?" to gauge the individual's response to technique application.

Consider how much change took place and how quickly in response to your work. Consider the overall stress level of the hands and the stress history of the individual. Compare the individual's rate of response to your expectations for similar patterns of stress such as age or stage of adaptation. Note whether or not change took place at the rate you expected.

Create a session plan for the individual. Outline the responses you observed and an assessment of the overall stress pattern. Give the individual an estimation of how much reflexology work will be required to achieve the goal that he or she has indicated.

The Integrated Session Plan Summary

The goal of the reflexologist is to efficiently and effectively apply technique. The question is, "How can the reflexologist best elicit the relaxation response so that the individual feels a change in stress level?" The integrated session combines observation, evaluation, application of technique, and communication.

Step One: Apply technique to the entire hand. Observe the hand for signs of alarm, adaptation, and / or exhaustion in the stress cues. Evaluate the stress cues to draw inferences about the hand, the reflex, and the body. Formulate a stress history by listening to the individual's comments and by asking questions.

Step Two: Apply technique to areas of emphasis during a second time through the hand. Review the stress cues and note the response to your technique application. Make inferences about how much technique application will be required to create a change in the stress pattern.

Step Three: Plan to create a successful relaxation strategy. Take stock of the individual's stress response, consider the individual's goals, note ongoing changes, and set a session strategy. Make an estimation of the commitment necessary to make the change desired.

The Length of the Session

A thirty to forty-five minute session is considered to be an appropriate length of time for technique application. A session that lasts more than an hour can overtax the client and create a reaction – flulike symptoms or discomfort caused by the release of toxins or waste products in the system.

Shorter session are applied with children. Shorter, more frequent sessions are utilized with the ill. A full-length session may overtax an already taxed body.

Summary Chart: Stress Inference & Technique Strategy

The goal of conditioning hand stress cues is to apply the technique strategy appropriate to the stress cue. The following is a reference chart of stress inferences and technique strategies appropriate to each. To use the chart, select the stress cue appropriate to the individual. Note the stress inference listed with the stress cue. Then, review the description of the technique strategy and consider it for appropriateness for application to the individual.

This chart should be used only as a guide and not as a diagnostic tool.

Stress Cue	Stress Inference	Technique Strategy
Visual Stress Cue		
Texture		
Puffiness	Puffiness over a broad area could indicate exhaustion. Over a small area, individual reports injury. Sharp sensitivity to technique application indicates current stress.	Note response. Apply more pressure if there is no sensitivity. Note response to repeated technique application. Avoid working and work the surrounding area if very sensitive.
Lacking tonus	Individual reports stress to stress-related musculo-skeletal problem.	Note response to repeated technique application.
Thickness	Individual reports occasional to recurring stress or stress-related condition. The depth of thickness indicates the length of time of adaptation to stress and amount of adaptation.	Begin with medium pressure. Note sensitivity. Note change of tonus in response to technique application.
Callousing	Individual reports work or hobby related activities that callus the hands.	Use medium to heavy pressure. Apply technique to the sides of the callousing with light to moderate pressure.
Color or Temperature	Individual reports occasional, isolated stress to chronic stress or stress-related condition or musculo-skeletal problem of the neck, upper back and/or shoulders. The more pronounced the color and the larger the area, the greater the impact of stress.	Apply technique. Observe any change in coloration. Note whether the hand changes in color or temperature by the end of the session.

188

Hand Feature		
Straightness of fingers	Individual reports recurring to chronic or stress-related musculo-skeletal problem. The angulation of fingers indicates the length of time of adaptation to stress and amount of adaptation to stress.	Apply movement techniques especially the walk down/pull against technique in a direction counter to the slant of the finger.
Joints	Individual reports recurring to chronic or stress-related condition. The thickness or redness indicates the length of time of adaptation to stress and amount of adaptation to stress.	Apply movement techniques especially encouraging movement with the side to side technique.
Scarring	Individual reports past injury. The size and color indicates amount of injury requiring adaptation to stress.	Apply technique around periphery of scarring and on scarring if not painful.
Color and shape of fingernails	See "Anatomy/Physiology," pages 48 - 50.	

Touch Stress Cue		
Puffiness	Sharp sensitivity to technique application indicates current stress. Individual reports current, occasional, or chronic stress or stress-related condition in the reflex area. Puffiness over a broad area could indicate general body stress.	Work from several directions to get a picture of the area. Use medium pressure. Use light pressure if the area is sensitive. If there is puffiness over the whole hand, use repeated passes of multiple finger walking on top of the hand. Note change. Be aware of the potential for hypersensitivity and blistering.
Lacking tonus	Individual reports current, occasional, or chronic stress or stress-related condition in a musculo-skeletal reflex area.	Apply multiple passes of technique over area.

Thickness	Individual reports recurring stress or stress-related condition. Thickness indicates an ongoing adaptation to stress over time. The thicker the tonus, the longer the length of time of adaptation and the more chronic the stress.	Work from several directions. Use moderate to heavy pressure. Thick tonus may be relatively insensitive at the beginning of technique application. Be aware that sensitivity may come out with repeated technique application. Note change. When you apply technique, does the tonus change and become less thick? More sensitive?
Hard Tonus	Individual reports long-term, chronic stress or stress-related condition. Does the individual report a continuous complaint, a past serious illness, or injury? The size and feel of the hard tonus varies from a small pea shape to a region of irregularly mounded hardness.	Use moderate to heavy pressure. Work on the area with caution and be aware of the potential for a sudden breakthrough of sensitivity. Expect sensitivity if the stress-related condition is active. Work the surrounding area and approach the sensitive area as sensitivity diminishes. Note change. Note difference in tonus of surrounding area.
Callousing	Individual reports work or hobby related activities that callus the hands.	Use medium to heavy pressure. Apply technique to the sides of the callousing with light to moderate pressure.
Stringiness	Individual reports current to occasional stress or stress-related condition if stringiness is sensitive and goes away with the application of pressure technique. Individual reports regular to chronic stress if the stringiness is sensitive, resistant to pressure technique, and does not go away.	Use light to moderate pressure. Expect sensitivity to come out with repeated technique application. Work surrounding area instead. Work the edges of the stringiness, moving closer and closer as the sensitivity diminishes.

Sensitivity Stress Cue

Be aware of the potential for overwork. An area feels overworked if it feels bruised to the touch. Avoid further work and, instead, work the surrounding area. "Ouch, that hurts" or withdrawal of the hand from you indicates a part of the hand that is sensitive, and that technique application is outside the individual's "comfort level." The area can be easily overworked, so avoid it.

Sensitivity	Individual reports current stress or stress-related condition or an active phase of a chronic problem or injury. The greater the sensitivity, the more the impact of the stress.	Note the individual's response to your technique application. "Ouch, that hurts good" is an indication that the area is sensitive but that the pressure level is within the individual's range of tolerance. Work from several directions to see if application from one direction is more sensitive than another. Do not work with an injured area.
Movement Stress Cues		
	Individual reports current stress or stress-related musculo-skeletal problem or an active phase of a chronic problem. The less the mobility, the more the impact of the stress.	Repeated application of movement techniques. Be aware of the potential for over-work.

CHAPTER 13

Tailoring the Session

When evaluating the hands, consider their background. Each pair of hands is a recorded history. The records are those of age, injury, and/or use. These considerations take into account the hands' experience - what they have been doing. A child's hand is evaluated differently form an adult's hand. The mechanic's hands exhibit characteristics different from those of a pianist. Each hand is evaluated in the context of its experience. Sports, hobbies, occupations and injuries all provide potential for stress and stress cues.

Eliciting and Noting Client Goals

Some clients readily volunteer such an extensive health history that its difficult to sort out exactly what's of most importance to them. Others - children especially - are not fluent in assessing their physical states and noting them. The goal is to listen when the information is volunteered, ask questions to elicit experience when its not, and to compare spoken comments to your observations.

Older Hands

Older hands have overpracticed and underpracticed the hands' activities over time. The net result is a change in what the hand is able to do. "Use it or lose" is particularly meaningful with older hands. Hands unable to move with flexibility can also develop into hands unable to maintain their owners' independent living status. Older hands need exercise, especially in directions of movement not frequently practiced. As a result, the application of movement techniques, especially those applied to the fingers and thumbs, are important. Fingers and thumbs provide the ability to manipulate buttons, zippers, and cooking utensils. A note of caution, however, is that older hands are set in their experiences. Work with older hands should not be pushed too far or too fast. Consider carefully the number of repetitions of technique application as well as the amount of pressure exerted.

Self-help is important. Show the client a simple, single technique that will produce results. We had one client who regained use of his hand enough to operate a remote control for the television set - an important step in his eyes. Another overcame arthritis of the hands on his own - so that he could apply reflexology work to his wife who had experienced a stroke. The sense of accomplishment, control, and hope for future positive actions has no replacement.

Children's Hands

Children's hands are involved in an educational process: learning how to handle the outside world, grasping an offered finger, holding a cup, drawing with a crayon. Learning to write is a primary communication skill developed in childhood. It is a usable skill, but it does place stresses on the hand. Further stressors are injury and growth.

The flexibility of childhood is deceptive. Children may "bounce

193

back" from injury and illness more easily than adults but there is no reason to believe that the best possible adjustment has been made. Memories of childhood linger with us, and so do the "dents." The physical memories of childhood form the basis of possible wear-and-tear patterns later in life. A finger slammed in a car door during childhood, for example, can result in a stiff joint into adulthood.

When working with children under the age of ten, the challenge to the reflexologist is to overcome the child's inherent short attention span. Five or ten minutes can be forever from the child's perspective. For infants, make the reflexology work into a game. Variations of "this little piggy" or applying reflexology techniques with the child's stuffed animal work well.

Children ask questions about what's going on. Explain that there are "owies" in their hands that you want to change to "feel good" areas.

Children are born with reflex areas that reflect stress, children undergo stressful situations and children encounter accidents. The growing pains of childhood are reflected in the endocrine reflex areas. Spills off the skateboard and other accidents are reflected in reflex areas of the skeletal system, especially the tail bone. Sports injuries and overuse are not uncommon with children. Find out what sport the child plays. Baseball or softball participation is reflected in stressed elbows, for example.

Self-help can and should be encouraged. Enlist the aid of the parents. A child who sees his or her parents using a sell-help reflexology technique is likely to pick up the habit. Our favorite story is the five-year old child who insisted that his parents turn the car around and return home so that he could retrieve "his" golf ball. (Not just any golf ball.) It wasn't until this point that his parents discovered he was using the golf ball on his hands to contend with his migraine headaches. It was a habit he had picked up at the babysitter's house, where she used a golf ball technique applied to the hands to help her sinus headaches.

The Stressed Adult

While some parts of the body are commonly impacted by stress - the endocrine glands, digestive system or lower back, it is important to recognize the individual's most stressed stress cue. While some joke about needing to store their stress somewhere, most stressed adults have at least one on-going stress-related health problem. For one business client always on the road, it was an old football heel injury. For another client, it was a wrenched neck. In working with stressed adults, alleviating the most stressful problem can provide an overall relaxation to reduce specific stress concerns. Then, further areas of stress can be approached.

Current Hand Injury

As usual in reflexology, the site of an injury is to be avoided. Determine if it is possible to work with the noninjured parts of the hand. Work with these areas of the hand will help the body adjust to the injury. It is a way of physically demonstrating that injury is present but that most parts of the hand are all right. Remember also that the foot is the referral area to the hand. Pinpoint for the client the area on the foot which reflects the hand injury. Determine if the client is able to comfortably apply self-help techniques to the foot.

Past Hand Injury

Determine the site of the injury and how the injury was created. In what direction was the hand or digit stretched and pulled? Consider this to be an indication of direction of stress. The muscles creating the opposite direction have been overly stressed and need to be relaxed. Also consider the movement technique application in the opposite direction. Consider the impact of other parts of the hand as a result of injury. For example, one injured joint in a finger changes the experiences of the entire finger. Movement technique is applied to the injured joint and also the other joints of the finger.

Repetitive Stress Injury

Two issues emerge from repetitive stress injury - the hand itself and the other parts of the body that create hand position. The neck, upper back, and arm all act to place the hand in its position of potential over use. Technique is applied to reflex areas relating to these body parts.

Current research in repetitive stress injury notes the importance of practicing directional movement of the hand. The hand is held in one position for too long thus resulting in injury. By practicing movement of the hand in directions other than those over-used, the hand relaxes.

In working with an individual with repetitive stress injury or the early stages of it, proceed slowly with your work. Any movement of the body of the should be done carefully. Stay in communication with the client and ask, "How does this feel? Is this too much?" Limit repetitions of directional movements.

CHAPTER 14

Tables of Disorders

The following table is a guide to suggested areas for evaluation and technique emphasis for various stress-related disorders. It should serve only as a guide and is not a diagnostic tool. The reflex areas are listed in descending order of importance.

AIDS	Lymphatic glands, Endocrine glands, Brain, Pancreas, Liver
Allergies	Adrenal glands, Reproductive glands, Pituitary
Alzheimer's	Brain, Brain stem, Kidneys, Endocrine glands
Anemia	Spleen, Liver, Thymus, Lymphatic
Angina-Pectoris	Heart, Adrenal glands, Chest, Lymphatic drain, Mid-back
Arthritis	Solar plexus, Kidneys, Adrenal glands, Thyroid
Asthma	Adrenal glands, Ileocecal valve, Solar plexus, Lungs
Back Disorders	Spine
Neck (Cervicals)	Neck, Tops of shoulders, Solar plexus

Lower Back (Lumbars)	Spine, Hip, Solar plexus, Knee / leg, Lymph / groin
Lower Back / Tailbone	Spine, Lumbar vertebrae
Bladder Disorders	Bladder, Kidney, Ureter tubes, Adrenal glands
Breast	Chest, Lymphatic glands, Pituitary
Bursitis	Shoulder, Adrenal glands, Colon
Cataracts	Eye / ear, Kidneys, Neck
Chronic fatigue syndrome	Adrenal glands, Pancreas
Colitis	Colon, Solar plexus, Adrenal glands
Constipation	Colon, Liver / gallbladder, Adrenal glands, Solar plexus, Lower back
Depression	Endocrine glands, Solar plexus, Pancreas, Head
Diabetes	Pancreas, Pituitary, Thyroid, Liver, Adrenal glands
Diverticulitis	Colon, Sigmoid colon, Solar plexus, Adrenal glands
Dizziness (Vertigo)	Eye / ear, Solar plexus
Earache	Eye / ear, Shoulder, Adrenal glands
Eczema	Endocrine glands, Solar plexus, Kidneys, Lymphatic glands
Emphysema	Lung, Ileocecal, Solar plexus, Colon
Eye Disorders	Eye, Neck, Kidneys
Fainting	Pituitary
Female Disorders	Uterus, Ovary, Fallopian tubes, Lower back
Fever	Pituitary
Fibromyalgeia	Lower back, Bladder, Tailbone, Solar plexus
Flatulence	Sigmoid colon, Solar plexus, Intestine
Glaucoma	Eye / ear, Neck, Kidneys
Gout	Kidneys, Corresponding body area

Hay Fever	Adrenal glands, Reproductive glands, Pituitary, Head / neck / sinus, Ileocecal valve
Headaches	Head / neck / sinus, Solar plexus, Tailbone and spine
Hearing Disorders	Eye / ear, Neck
Heart Attack	Heart / lung, Adrenal glands, Sigmoid colon
Hemorrhoids	Tailbone, Hip region, Lower back, Sigmoid colon, Solar plexus
Hernia	Lymphatic / groin, Lower back, Hip, Adrenal glands
Hiatal Hernia	Solar plexus, Adrenal glands
Hip Disorders	Lymphatic / groin, Hip region, Hip / back / sciatic, Knee / leg, Lower back
Hypertension	Solar plexus, Adrenal glands, Kidneys, Pituitary, Liver, Thyroid
Hypoglycemia	Pancreas, Pituitary, Thyroid, Liver, Adrenal glands
Impotence	Prostate, Testes, Solar plexus
Infertility	Uterus, Ovaries, Groin / Lymphatic glands / Fallopian tubes
Kidney disorders	Kidney, Ureter tubes, Bladder
Kidney Stones	Kidneys, Ureter tubes, Bladder
Macular degeneration	Head / Neck / Sinus, Eye
Menopause	Uterus, Ovaries
Menstruation	Uterus, Ovaries, Lower back
Migraine	Tailbone, Head / Neck
Numbness in the Finger-tips	Neck
Pain	Solar plexus, Adrenal glands
Paralysis	Eye / ear, Entire body of the foot, Neck, Spine, Top of head

Phlebitis	Liver, Adrenal glands, Kidneys, Lymphatic / groin, Knee / leg
Premenstrual syndrome	Uterus, Ovaries, Solar plexus, Groin / Lymphatic glands / Fallopian tubes
Prostate Disorders	Prostate, Testes
Psoriasis	Kidneys, Thyroid, Adrenal glands, Pituitary
Sciatica	Hip / sciatic, Lymphatic / groin, Lower back / tailbone, Knee / leg
Shingles	Spine, Solar plexus
Shoulder Disorders	Shoulder, Neck, Midback, Arm, Tops of the shoulders, Digestive system
Skin Disorders	Reproductive glands, Kidneys, Thyroid, Adrenal glands, Pituitary
Sore Throat	Neck, Adrenal glands, Lymphatic
Stroke	Top of head, Head, Eye / ear, Solar plexus, Spine
Tinnitis	Eye / ear, Neck, Adrenal glands, Shoulder
Tonsillitis	Neck. Lymphatic, Adrenal glands
Toothache	Head / Neck / Sinus
Ulcer	Stomach (if affected), Solar plexus, Diaphragm, Adrenal glands, Colon, Endocrine glands
Whiplash	Neck, Lung, Spine

CHAPTER 15

Charts Summary

Foot Reflexology Chart

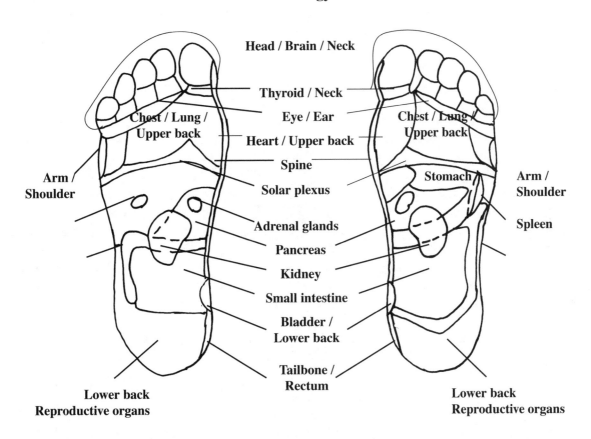

Head / Brain / Neck

Thyroid / Neck

Chest / Lung / Upper back

Eye / Ear

Heart / Upper back

Chest / Lung / Upper back

Spine

Stomach

Arm / Shoulder

Solar plexus

Arm / Shoulder

Adrenal glands

Spleen

Pancreas

Kidney

Small intestine

Bladder / Lower back

Tailbone / Rectum

Lower back Reproductive organs

Lower back Reproductive organs

Touch Stress Cues

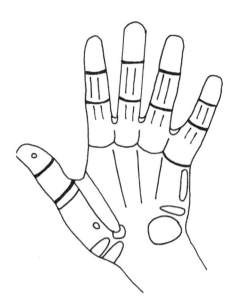
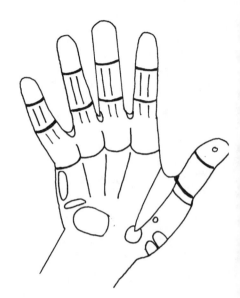

Temperature:
Hot
Cold
Perspiring

Texture:
Puffiness
Thickness
Lack of tonus
Hard tonus
Callousing

Sensitivity

Visual Stress Cues

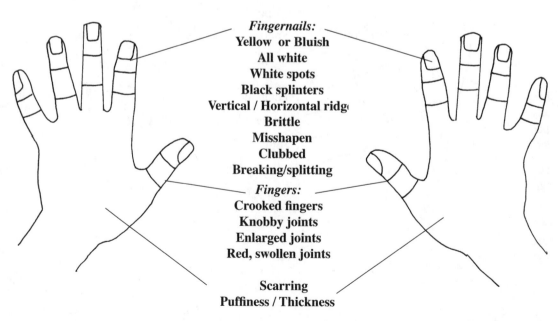

Fingernails:
Yellow or Bluish
All white
White spots
Black splinters
Vertical / Horizontal ridge
Brittle
Misshapen
Clubbed
Breaking/splitting

Fingers:
Crooked fingers
Knobby joints
Enlarged joints
Red, swollen joints

Scarring
Puffiness / Thickness

Hand Reflexology Chart

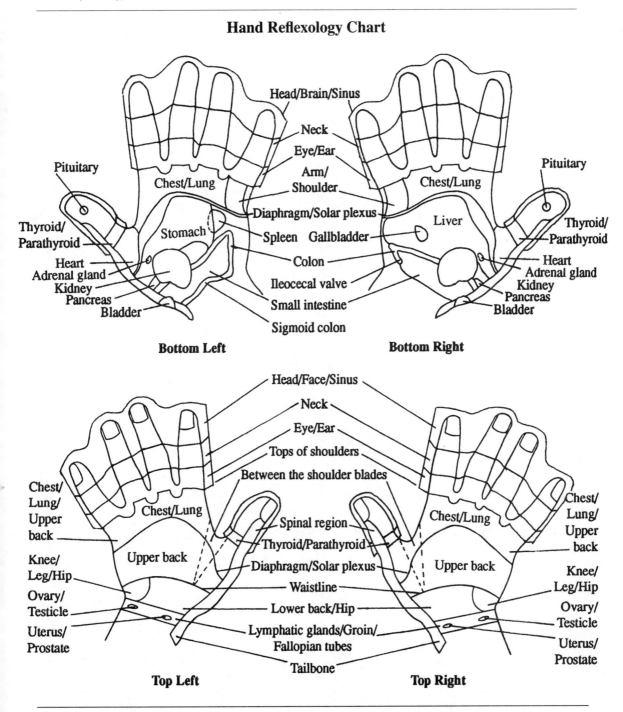

Head/Brain/Sinus
Neck
Eye/Ear
Arm/Shoulder
Pituitary
Chest/Lung
Diaphragm/Solar plexus
Thyroid/Parathyroid
Stomach
Spleen Gallbladder
Liver
Chest/Lung
Pituitary
Thyroid/Parathyroid
Heart
Adrenal gland
Kidney
Pancreas
Bladder
Colon
Ileocecal valve
Small intestine
Sigmoid colon
Heart
Adrenal gland
Kidney
Pancreas
Bladder

Bottom Left   **Bottom Right**

Head/Face/Sinus
Neck
Eye/Ear
Tops of shoulders
Between the shoulder blades
Chest/Lung/Upper back
Chest/Lung
Spinal region
Thyroid/Parathyroid
Diaphragm/Solar plexus
Chest/Lung
Chest/Lung/Upper back
Knee/Leg/Hip
Upper back
Waistline
Upper back
Knee/Leg/Hip
Ovary/Testicle
Lower back/Hip
Ovary/Testicle
Uterus/Prostate
Lymphatic glands/Groin/Fallopian tubes
Uterus/Prostate
Tailbone

Top Left   **Top Right**

Index

Information Please

Join internationally recognized authors Kevin and Barbara Kunz in:
- Integrating reflexology into the medical community and your community
- Boosting your reflexology knowledge and skills
- Expanding your professinal horizons
- Communicate your reflexology experiences

Please send me information about:

_____ Reflexology Training
_____ Hand Reflexology Curriculum (Instructor Manual, Overlays)
_____ Assessment for Reflexologists Curriculum(Instructor Manual, Overlays)
_____ 200-hour Reflexology Curriculum Package (Instructor Mauals, Overlays)

Please send me the complimentary newsletter *Reflexions:*

_____ On-line
_____ By mail

Please place me on your mailing list:

_____ On-line
_____ By mail

_____ **Please sign me up for the on-line Reflexology Community**

Name _____

Address _____

City _____ **State** _____ **Zip code**_____

email address _____
I maintain a Web site at _____

Join us on-line at www.foot-reflexologist.com

Order Blank

Books and Charts by Kevin and Barbara Kunz

____*The Complete Guide to Foot Reflexology (Revised)* ($16.95) .... _____

Postage and Handling $2.50

____**Hand and Foot Reflexology, A Self-Help Guide** ($13)..................... _____

Postage and Handling $2.50

____ **Hand Reflexology Workbook (Revised)** ($16.95) .... _____

Postage and Handling $2.50

____ **The Parent's Guide to Reflexology** ($16.00) .... _____

Postage and Handling $2.50

____ **Medical Applications of Reflexology**: Findings in Research about Safety, Efficacy, Mechanisms of Action and Cost-Effectiveness of Reflexology ($29.95, 32 pages) _____

Postage and Handling $2.50

____ *My Reflexologist Says Feet Don't Lie* ($9.95)........................ .... ____

Postage and Handling $2.50

____**Foot and Hand Reflexology laminated charts in color** ($4.95, 3 1/2" x 6") _____

TOTAL _____

____ My check or money order is enclosed.

____ Please accept my order and charge my account with: ___Master Card ___Visa

Charge Card Number __ __ __ __ - __ __ __ __ - __ __ __ __ - __ __ __ __

Signature_____ Expiration date_____

Name _____

Address _____

City _____ **State** _____ **Zip code**_____

All prices are U. S. currency and subject to change.
Note: Actual postage charges added to overseas orders.

Mail your order to Reflexology Research, P. O. Box 35820, Albuquerque, NM 87176

Phone: 505-344-9392, FAX: 505-344-0246, email: footc@aol.com

Order on-line at www.reflexology-research.com